For Freddie

For Freddie

A MOTHER'S FINAL GIFT TO HER SON

RACHAEL BLAND

The royalties from this book (2% of the purchase price) will be donated to Breast Cancer Now, a charity registered in England and Wales (no. 1160558), Scotland (SC045584) and Isle of Man (no. 1200). From 1 April 2019 Breast Cancer Now's new registered name will be Breast Cancer Care and Breast Cancer Now.

MICHAEL O'MARA BOOKS LIMITED

First published in Great Britain in 2019 by
Michael O'Mara Books Limited
9 Lion Yard
Tremadoc Road
London SW4 7NQ

A CIP catalogue record for this book is available from the British Library.

Papers used by Michael O'Mara Books Limited are natural, recyclable products
made from wood grown in sustainable forests. The manufacturing processes
conform to the environmental regulations of the country of origin.

ISBN: 978-1-78929-132-2 in hardback print format
ISBN: 978-1-78929-135-3 in ebook format
ISBN: 978-1-78929-139-1 in audiobook format

With heartfelt thanks to *HuffPost UK* for granting permission to reproduce the
introduction, which was first published on 4 September 2018, the day before
Rachael died. With thanks also to the *Sun* for granting permission to reproduce
Richard Bacon's tribute, and the *The Times* for Deborah James' tribute.

First plate section credits: page 15 and 16 (top left): Sian Trenberth
Second plate section credits: page 30 (bottom) *Stylist*; page 31: BBC Images

1 2 3 4 5 6 7 8 9 10

Printed in the UK by CPI Group (UK) Ltd, Croydon, CR0 4YY
Deisgned and typeset by K.DESIGN, Winscombe, Somerset

www.mombooks.com

FOR OUR GIRL, RACHAEL

Love, Steve and Freddie

ACKNOWLEDGEMENTS

And so it falls to me to thank some incredibly important people, not just for being a part of this book and for contributing stories, pictures or tributes, but for all the support they have given Rachael over so many years.

To her dear mother Gayna, her late father David, her brother Matthew, his partner Kirsty, to Matthew's children, Emily and William, and her wider family, Rachael cherished you all, and your love and guidance helped to grow and nurture the person who we all fell in love with.

To my mum, my dad, my sister Claire, brother-in-law Mark and their children, Imogen, Matilda and Barney, thank you for making Rachael such an important part of our family. She loved you all very much.

Thank you to Rachael's Welsh girls, who became her London girls with a few additions, in particular her most treasured friend Jo; to her cherished uni girls with whom she spent some of her very happiest years and to her NCT gang, in particular her dear friend Rachael, who time after time dropped everything to be with her.

To everyone at 5 Live, and right across the wider broadcasting world, who supported Rachael both in her day-to-day work and in the creation of the amazing *You, Me and the Big C* podcast, thank you.

Thank you also to Lauren, Debs, Mike and Al for helping to turn her podcast idea into the glorious, life-changing juggernaut it became. To everyone who listened to that podcast or read Rachael's blog, thank you. Your messages carried her through some dark times and gave her more comfort than you'll ever know.

This book features contributions from some of the most important people in Rachael's professional life, so to everyone who jumped at the chance to contribute – Richard, Tony, Jonno, Emma B, Shelagh, Chris, Dermot, Greg, Emma A, Mark, Rachel – thank you so much. Your words make us all even more proud of our girl, if indeed that was even possible. And on the topic of the book, I have to thank Heather at HHB Agency and Nicki at Michael O'Mara Books for their passion and drive to see this book become what you hold in your hands now.

Thank you so very much to all the incredible doctors and nurses who did so much for Rachael, and thank you too to Claire and Rich Paxman, who went above and beyond to make sure Rachael kept her fabulous hair. You made such a difference and I'll never be able to thank you enough.

And lastly to Rachael. From me. Thank you for everything. Falling in love with you, marrying you, having and raising Freddie with you, and even going through this awful disease with you has been the greatest honour and privilege of my life. I wouldn't change a thing about the past seven years and Freddie and I will love you, miss you and hold you in our hearts forever.

With the help of this book, we'll keep your light shining for many, many years yet.

Thank you all,

Steve x

CONTENTS

INTRODUCTION

27 AUGUST 2018

'I'm sorry Rachael, it's back and it's incurable.' From the moment you're diagnosed with breast cancer, or any type of cancer, they're the words you really don't want to hear. That's why you and your oncologists spend all your time working as hard as possible to stop the cancer spreading. But sometimes it is just too aggressive, and nothing can stem its growth.

My D-Day call – I jokingly refer to it as 'Death-Day'– came back in April 2018, while I was out playing with my three-year-old son, Freddie. Hearing those words ripped the air right out of my lungs and I had to lean against a wall to steady myself. Holding in the huge sobs I knew were coming, I just needed to get home and call my surgeon in peace with my husband at my side. On the short journey back, I wept and kept saying to him, 'I'm so sorry'.

This cancer is growing wildly throughout my body and I can't put that down to anyone else but me. It's a terrible feeling that my body has some role in putting my family through the pain I know awaits them. As ever, I knew I would share this news on our podcast, *You,*

Me and the Big C, and my blog. The whole sharing process has been very cathartic. It's been a real support to know that people have found them so helpful through their treatment, but in a selfish way they've helped me just as much.

When I was eventually ready to talk about my diagnosis, as I recalled those feelings of devastation, I found myself crying on the podcast for the first time. In return I received such an outpouring of love and grief from family, friends, acquaintances and strangers alike, it was quite overwhelming. I was sent so many beautiful messages.

When you are in my position – knowingly approaching the end of your life at just forty years old, with a husband you adore with all your heart and a three-year-old son you love so much that if you looked at him too long your heart could burst – you need two major things to get you through. Hope. And denial.

It is as a mother that I have to deploy my strongest skills of denial. I'm too scared to ask the doctors how long I've got left – it would be a guesstimate number that would hang over me. So, we make plans, knowing it's not very long.

If I were to release all my feelings about leaving my precious, beautiful Freddie behind, I wouldn't be able to enjoy the rest of my time on this earth. So, I tuck them away, graciously accept every little hug, squeeze, cuddle and utterance of 'I love you so much, Mummy' and try not to let him see it break my heart.

I have written my memoir, *For Freddie*, which is a collection of all those stories your parents tell you over the years from their point of view, mixed in with all the advice they give you. I'd only known Steve for such a short period of time before we married – I feel there's so much Freddie needs to know from my point of view and in my voice. And I think I best get my personality down on paper.

I hope the book will leave an imprint of my love behind for the rest of his life. So he can be sure how very much I love him.

Love,
Rachael x

Chapter 1

A FEW OF MY FAVOURITE THINGS (AND SOME I CAN'T STAND)

'Raindrops on roses and whiskers on kittens' … these are not actually my favourite things but a line sung by a great actress called Julie Andrews from a song in a cheesy movie, which seems a good place to start the book. I LOVE a rubbish movie Freddie, really love them. If it's a musical to boot, then even better. This particular one is called *The Sound of Music* and was made in 1965, which to you reading this will seem like ancient times but incredibly it was just thirteen years before Mummy was born. I hope it's still popular now. I think you could even sit down and watch it with Daddy as it has the crucial World War Two element that he loves.

If a film critic says a film is rubbish, then I know I'm going to love it. This may be down to my slightly stubborn nature which I can see you have inherited already (that's my boy!). I don't like to be told what to do and what to like. And that's a good thing; you make up your own mind in life. Autonomy is important, you have the intelligence to not just follow the crowd. Let's add to the list of movies Mummy has watched a thousand times, all the classics are there … like *Pretty Woman*. I loved the fairy-tale aspect of the story and even wrote a piece of coursework on how it linked into the fairy-tale themes identified by Russian theorist Vladimir Propp (look him up!). There is nothing wrong with dreaming of a fairy tale as long as you are active and not passive and put plans into practice. *Pretty Woman* was made in 1990 and even now in 2018 it has become a little un-PC. Feminism has moved on in leaps and bounds, and the idea that a woman needs a good man to rush in and save her is somewhat outdated. But I still like to believe in a story with a happy ending, whether the prince rescues the princess or she charges out of the castle herself!

I am also a huge fan of any kind of rom-com, *Love Actually*-esque, feel-good film. The clue is in the description – I like to watch things on TV that make me feel good and happy because that's just a nice way to feel, isn't it? I haven't watched a horror film since I was about fifteen – they would stay with me. There's enough horror and misery in the world not to add to it with fictional accounts in my honest opinion! Though I do admire people who have the resilience of mind to happily sit through a terrifying two hours at the cinema then skip home happily untouched by what they have seen. I love a comedy, as I love to laugh. Laughing is good for your very soul. I hope you laugh as much in the future as you do now. You currently find yourself and other things so funny that you frequently laugh until you're sick! I love to see you this happy and discovering your own sense of humour. Always keep that, let's just hope the vomiting bit settles or that could get annoying on nights out with friends.

Other things I love … the colour yellow. It's just a happy colour, isn't it? It's sunshine and spring and flowers. It makes me feel happy and serene. I have been known to overuse it. The time in my second year at Cardiff University when I painted my radiator and the door to the utility room (I didn't have a window, more uni tales to come later) a very vivid shade of yellow was probably a mistake. But you can't go wrong with a bit of yellow clothing. You've had plenty of yellow tops in your wardrobe and you're only three.

That's another thing I love to do – shop. I'm a terrible overspender; your dad is too. We're very much of the 'buy it now, worry about paying for it later' ethos. I had hoped to instil in you a better sense of saving for things as you grow up and being sensible with your money but I'm not sure that would have panned out very well as I filled your wardrobe with way too many bits from Boden twice a year. But you never know, sometimes these things skip a generation, and you won't be vying for cupboard space with Daddy to house your shoe collections. He's the only man I've ever known to own more shoes than me. But again, it all comes down to what makes you happy and if that is a shoe collection to rival Imelda Marcos (again – one to look up on Wikipedia) then so be it.

You'll note my frequent references to what are now probably defunct research tools – that is the journalist in me. I've loved the news and knowing what is going on in the world. It is always good to be informed. It puts you ahead of the game. At its very basic level my love for news is pure nosiness and being the first in with the gossip! I decided fairly early on that I wanted to be a broadcast journalist and just went for it. I was lucky that I knew what I wanted to do and could focus. If you have that too then brilliant, but if you can't decide or nothing seems to grab you, then just head out into the world and experience things and you'll find your path. It all comes back to that autonomy of thought and knowing yourself and what you want out of life. If that takes years then fine; if you know when you're ten, great. But remember you are here to make yourself and those around you happy, so always keep that in mind.

At school I hated all the team sports, though with hindsight I wish I had participated more. I loved long-distance running and swimming. I was good at both but never excelled and I always wanted for you to do as much sport as you could if you are that way inclined. I suspect you will be, as you currently have boundless energy and love running around outside and climbing and jumping. Plus, you've got your daddy's long legs and if you listen to him he could have been a pro in most sports (only joking, Daddy). I know he's going to have you on the season-ticket list at Liverpool FC, but don't feel you have to be a footballer. You find a sport that makes you happy and do your best at it.

I was very much a couch potato for a time after leaving university until I found running again and joined a triathlon club. I loved the variety of swimming, cycling and running. I was never the fastest but I always just liked to race myself on the way round, setting little targets and personal bests. Then there was a halcyon period exercise-wise where I ran the London Marathon three years in a row between 2010 and 2012. First and last I ran with injuries in a still respectable four and a half hours or so. The middle year was my one sub-four hour (the holy grail of amateur marathon running) which I think I achieved by accident. Having studiously kept a steady pace with my running GPS watch, I lost signal in a tunnel around Canary Wharf somewhere. I thought my pace was dropping off, so in my usual belligerent way I stepped it up. As I emerged from all the high-rise buildings, I suddenly realized I was running much faster than I had trained for, but I couldn't stop my legs turning over for fear of slowing to a stop. So, on I carried to the finish like the girl in 'The Red Shoes', my little feet going as fast as they could. And I miraculously crossed the line in three hours, fifty-two minutes and fifty-three seconds ... you never forget your best marathon time! And it again goes to show that sometimes your best results can be achieved when you don't follow the plan.

Doing more exercise and getting some strength in my legs let me discover one of the great loves of my life – skiing! I hope by now that Daddy has taken you and taught you and you love it. There is nothing in life so good as breathing in fresh mountain air as you fly down the piste looking at the beautiful snowy landscape around you. Snow is just magical and can turn the dullest of vistas into the most spectacular. It's the best kind of holiday – always so social with lots of friends, everyone in the mood to chat. You cross paths (hopefully not on the piste!) with lots of different nationalities and all topped off with yummy food and drink and lots of fabulous clothes. What is not to like!?

Learning to ski was another one of those things I did to prove people wrong. My university boyfriend was a very good skier but would never take me with him as he feared I'd hold him and his friends up. So, I went and booked a trip with my friends Uma and Rae and off we went to Châtel in France for a weekend, where I was determined to come away a top downhill skier! I of course didn't, but I persisted and went as much as I could the following years. I was very much of the 'point down the mountain, don't look at the colour of the piste' school of skiing! I tried to get a little technique in there and I'm proud to say I eventually became a good skier. It's also taken me to the age of forty to be proud to say that kind of thing. I grew up thinking modesty was the best approach and doing the typical British thing of playing down my skills and batting away compliments. But actually, you can talk about your achievements and skills and be proud of what you can do without being seen as conceited or arrogant. Always try … or you'll never know if you can do it. And as my good friend Uma said (on that holiday, I believe), 'Reach for the stars and you may just end up hitting the top of the lamp post'.

As promised, a list of things I hate … but let's not spend too much time on these as they're a waste of energy! They include … spiders –

it's the crawling! It's totally irrational as in this country they can't hurt you, but then that's the thing about fear – it's often irrational. This has developed into a fear of most insects – moths, flies, daddy-long-legs. Wasps! What is their point in life? However, this doesn't extend to bees – they are friendly and do the work of spreading pollen and making honey and I love a bit of honey. We've just been trying to rescue some tired ones in the garden with sugar and water on a spoon which you have loved.

I'm always late, so I hate it when people are on time! Traits-wise, I can't stand arrogance; people who like the sound of their own voices too much and those without empathy. I can already see you are full of empathy. I had some pain the other day and you dashed straight for your medical kit and checked me with your stethoscope and thermometer. You are so caring and can read people's feelings. These are excellent personality traits to have inherited – I say this because they are from me.

Chapter 2

WHEN MUMMY MET DADDY

N ow here's a tale of two sides, Freddie! It was relatively late in life that your daddy and I crossed paths – we both agreed that we wished we'd met sooner and spent more of our formative years together, but sometimes you have to wait for the best things in life. And every moment, every second of our meeting and what followed I believe was mapped out to lead us to have you … our beautiful, perfect, fun-loving Fred.

I was thirty-three and Daddy was thirty-one in 2011 when we both worked at the BBC on Radio 5 Live. This was a year of big change at the BBC as a large section of the corporation that had been based at the wonderful, iconic Television Centre – with its years of historic broadcasts and the voices of the most famous entertainers of all time emanating from its walls – was to move to a new home at MediaCityUK in Salford, more than 200 miles away. It was a time of great upheaval for many of my colleagues, but I saw it as an opportunity to get more work in the daytime (I was at the time the 'late newsreader' on air until 1 a.m. – very antisocial) and to make a fresh start. Most of my London friends were settling down and getting married. I was single, didn't own any property and so it was an easy and exciting move to head north for a new challenge.

It was a very social time. We moved up programme team by programme team, with me being in the first group. I was in fact (*humble brag klaxon*) the first voice to broadcast live from the BBC's new MediaCityUK studios. At the time I was working with Tony Livesey (one of the nicest men in broadcasting – you *can* get to the top while remaining a good person) and the honour was meant to be his. Then they decided to start with the news and I whisked the historic moment away from him!

By the time Daddy's team from the 5 Live Breakfast show arrived on the scene I had been happily settled into my lovely new little rental flat in Hale in Cheshire for a couple of months. Making the move encouraged me to get out and socialize as much as possible to build up a new network of friends. I am a natural introvert – quite unusual for a journalist, but as I've said already I never like to stick to the norms – so sometimes I need a push in the right direction with social events as I find that while I have a wonderful time, all the talking and keeping up conversation can sap my natural energy.

A night out was arranged to welcome the Breakfast team and I was dragged along by my friend Lucy to the Rain Bar in the centre of Manchester to hang out. Then I had my 'cheesy movie moment' as I locked eyes with your daddy across the bar and thought, 'Hello, who's the handsome new chap they've signed up to the Breakfast team?!' As it later transpired, he had already been working at 5 Live for over a year and we'd actually worked together when I had stood in to present the *Weekend Breakfast* show. Ooops! There's another bit of 'do as I say and not as I do' for you; always walk around the world with your head up and your eyes open. Do not miss an opportunity that could be staring you in the face.

By all accounts, I think Daddy already had a crush on me at this point and we could have got together way sooner had I just been more aware.

Anyway, back to the Rain Bar. We chatted a bit over a G&T or two and I was thrilled to find out this handsome, tall stranger (as we've already deduced NOT actually a stranger) was going to be moving in two minutes away from me in Hale with my friends Mike and Garth. What fortune! So vague plans were made to pop over once they were all ensconced in their new house in a few weeks' time.

The day came and I nearly cancelled. I was just back from the wedding of my other friend Lucy and her husband Mark at a beautiful house in Wales where the cocktails were too free-flowing. Me and my old friend, your Auntie Jo, had woken up on sofas in the wedding house with vague memories of jumping in the indoor pool and doing swimming races at about 4 a.m. After a long journey back north, the last thing I felt like doing was socializing with my new neighbours, but something made me go. Your daddy was the one of the three chaps I knew least, but somehow we spent the whole night talking and found we had so much in common. I knew that night that after thirty-three years I had found the man I wanted to marry. For so long I had heard the old adage 'when you know, you know' and I never knew … until that moment, when you just know! It's like the other half of your soul that's been missing, and then slots in like the last jigsaw piece and you can relax … 'Ah, there you are.'

A couple of days later we went to the BBC 5 Live big Christmas bash together. I met Daddy at Hale train station with Garth, unsure of whether a kiss on the cheek to say hello was appropriate for this man I had just met but already knew I would marry. As I recall, I went in for the peck on the cheek, as I've always been a hugger. Better to 'over' emote in a situation than 'under' in my opinion!

The Christmas party passed in a blur. There were drinks, perhaps some pizza, a lot of merry colleagues and dodgy Christmas dancing. But again, I had that movie moment where all around us seemed to revolve quietly and all I cared about was keeping my seat next to Daddy before any other girls moved in to chat to him. This was noted by a few colleagues in the following days – a lot of 'You and Steve were getting on VERY WELL at the party … nudge nudge'.

There had still been no kiss, no particular understanding between us (that sounds so very Jane Austen!) but we knew. I effectively made the first move by adding your daddy as a friend on Facebook – the equivalent of asking him out in those days! And then, just like in every good story, came a time of enforced separation with the arrival of Christmas which was followed for me by a nine-day ski holiday over New Year. Now I've already discussed my love of skiing but this now seemed like an unnecessarily long time to go for. It would mean almost three weeks apart when we hadn't even really got together. We kept in touch by text all over this time, but I got quite jealous when your daddy said he'd had the mistletoe out in church on Christmas Day. I thought he was trying to make me jealous but he's just not the sort of guy to play mind games – it turned out the kisses were mainly doled out to the mothers of his friends!

I had taken my brother, your Uncle Matthew, skiing with me and he was quite a lot to handle on a night out at the time! Your daddy managed to talk me down from throttling him after he gave me the fright of my life when I lost him on New Year's Eve and he decided to spend the night down the mountain with some new friends (see skiing is very social!) and came back bouncing off the walls at 9 a.m. insisting on coming out skiing for the day. There's another sage bit of advice – don't mix alcohol and skiing, you need to have your wits about you to avoid injury. A beer at lunchtime is fine, then wait until dinner for the wine!

So, through those few weeks of texting we both knew that when I arrived home, getting together was a fait accompli. We had spent a lot of time chatting about our love of onesies, we were always big fans of comfies! So, when Daddy headed over to see me the night I got home, I answered the door in my pink-and-navy Jack Wills Christmas onesie with a fridge full of cheese and wine, and that was that. We had our first kiss in the lounge that evening, then spent the next two months or so putting on some 'happy fat' via the cheese, wine and general loved-up-ness. So much so that by the time we booked our first holiday together in the March – St Anton skiing – I had to buy a new pair of ski trousers a size up, as the ones I wore in January were too tight! But it was worth it for the falling in love over cheese and wine.

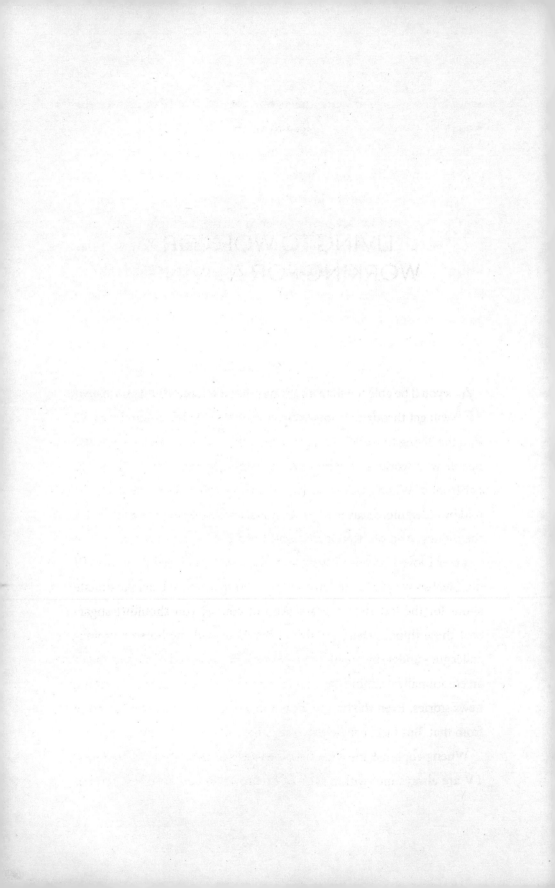

Chapter 3

LIVING TO WORK OR WORKING FOR A LIVING?

As you'll be able to tell from the number of mentions that my career will get throughout this book, for me this big life conundrum fell into the 'living to work' to category. That is not to say I am one of those people who works all the hours God sends and gets paid a mint for it. Far from it. When I was making my way into journalism I kept getting told by older, more seasoned professionals not to expect to go into it for the money. And oh, were they right! But I carried on in my pursuit of a career I loved because I truly have thoroughly enjoyed doing what I do. I feel so very lucky to have found a job that I have been passionate about for the last twenty years. And of course, you shouldn't sugar-coat these things. There are days where I cursed the boss or various colleagues under my breath or just arrived home wiped out at the end of an emotionally draining day of reading some of the most heartbreaking news stories. Even the best work is still work – there's no getting away from that. But I feel privileged to say I have loved my career.

When people ask me what I do, the words broadcasting, radio, news, TV are always met with a raise of eyebrows and an air of excitement and hey, it's nice when people are interested in what you do. It's always a good 'in' on a conversation. I tell people that I never feel like my job is a 'real' job. There is not enough daily grind to it, I don't feel like the work is hard enough because I enjoy it so much. It's not like working in an office. I sit next to an 'on-air' studio every day, popping in and out to read the news, never knowing which celebrity I will find sitting in there one minute or, even better, someone I've never heard of the next, telling a story across the airwaves that is just so gripping that I don't want to leave my seat and go back to my desk and miss a word.

That's the business we are in, and what I think makes radio such a special medium. We are that friendly voice in the background you can have on while going about the tasks of daily life. You get on with the household chores and we keep you informed about the daily news events, tell you some funny stories of our own and let our guests tell you theirs. Over the last couple of years, I have done more presenting; weirdly, the nightmare of having cancer and wanting to share my feelings about it taught me how to be more open and honest and give more of myself on air. Sometimes, my darling, timing in life is just a bit of an arse! But as my dad, your Grandad Hodges, used to say, 'What can't be cured, must be endured'.

It was around the age of fifteen or so that I really decided I wanted to be a broadcast journalist. I've always enjoyed writing and again weirdly, for someone who was very shy as a youngster I liked the sound of my own voice! At first glance that would seem at odds with the traits I said I disliked earlier. But this was not about me wanting to hear my own voice chatting away about myself, I just loved to read out loud! I was a prolific reader of books when I was younger, mostly about ponies and horses. I would pick them up from the school book fairs or spend any pocket money on the latest releases at John Menzies when we went into

Cardiff shopping on a Saturday. Whenever they went around English class looking for someone to read the next chapter, while most of the class tried to hide behind their books I would always want it to be me. In primary-school plays I was often chosen as the narrator. It probably should have been a lot more obvious to me what I wanted to do much sooner!

I did some work experience via a friend of my mum, your Grandma, at the then HTV Wales news studios in Culverhouse Cross. I was still super-shy at this point but followed the reporters around wide-eyed on their jobs as I went out with the cameramen, watched them film their pieces and then come back and sit in an edit suite to turn them into an item for the evening news. My overriding feeling was one of rising excitement as I thought a) this looks like a lot of fun and b) this looks pretty easy (NB: in the interests of all my colleagues I leave behind, the job is REALLY, REALLY hard and they should all be paid more!).

There followed more work experience at Red Dragon Radio in Cardiff before I followed what I thought was the 'safe' route in through academia. In 1996 I went to Cardiff University to do its Journalism, Film and Broadcasting degree before doing a postgraduate degree in Broadcast Journalism at the University of Central Lancashire in 2000. This sounds like a smooth transition but don't be fooled, life is never that simple. At this time came my first lesson in 'if at first you don't succeed then try, try again'. I had wanted to stay on to do the postgrad course at Cardiff. I had thought this was my destiny. But as I've mentioned before I was pretty shy at this stage still and not great at talking in groups … and the interview for the course? It was a group one obviously! And who was last to speak – yep, your mummy. And who had worked herself up into a terrible sweat about what to say to introduce herself and impress the tutors – YES, your mummy. By the time my turn came I was so nervous I could barely string a sentence together. I stumbled my way through a load of old rubbish and glanced down at the notes one of the lecturers was writing on the table right next to me: 'Not very lucid' he had jotted down. Now it doesn't take a genius to work out that's not the kind of trait they were looking for in their best journalism students. I cried and cried when the letter came to say I hadn't got on the course. But I quickly learnt that when these knock-backs come along, you've got to have a bit of a cry, let it all out, pick yourself up, dust yourself down and put yourself out there again.

Twenty-year-old me, who was terrified to speak in public yet desperate to be on the radio, seems a world away from forty-year-old me, who you have to turn the volume down on because she's banging on about herself on the *You, Me and the Big C* podcast again! The lesson I guess here, my Fred, is that if you're of a sensitive disposition like your mummy, which I can see you already are, then you've got to try and develop a thick skin, try not to take things to heart too much, feel and grieve your disappointments because not everything can go your way in life, then get back out there again and carry on living. As I now know only too well, you only get one chance at life so grab every opportunity you can and keep on trying. The tutors on the course seemed rather pleased with themselves when they revealed they'd turned down TV news legend Huw Edwards for a place, so really what did they know anyway?

I have spent most of my career at the BBC and it is a public corporation I love so much. I'm not sure if it will exist in the same form for you now but I know its mark will still be around. Back when there were only four TV channels, it was affectionately known as 'Auntie' and while, like that other great and I hope still publicly funded institution the NHS, it has many faults and areas for improvements in the way it is run, it has provided a brilliant service informing, educating and entertaining the nation over the years. I am so very proud to have played a small part in that.

I started my very first broadcasts outside of the big walls of the BBC, though, at a tiny new start-up station above a pub in Bridgend in South Wales, aptly named Bridge FM! Less salubrious surroundings than those of the famous BBC Television Centre which I would eventually frequent. Through my work experience contacts they were given my name, I turned up for a chat and then suddenly found myself employed as a part-time newsreader on the station. I walked away in a state of shock and about to partake in my first bit of 'winging it'. Had I read the news before? Only onto a cassette player at home. I needed to set up the news-desk contacts and working practices – uh, I had a mini-Filofax?? But I turned up and read my news in an accent far more Welsh than the one I ended up with.

Because it was a small new commercial station it was a great place to make all my mistakes (okay, okay, 5 Live texters – some of them!), like the time your grandma called me approximately two seconds after I finished a news bulletin to tell me the Turkish capital was pronounced ANK-ara and not an-CARA. This of course was not my most embarrassing mistake on air. That came much later at 5 Live, *obviously* on network radio, when I got a little confused over some last-minute breaking news about a band called 'The xx' winning the 2010 Mercury Prize for their debut album entitled *xx*. 'XX' is a shorthand we radio journalists often use when we're waiting to hear the name for something to add into a script at the last minute. Cue me twice thinking the producer had forgotten to write the winner's details in the script. Cue much hilarity from all the listeners who'd actually heard of The xx! If you Google it and the Radio Fail website still exists, you can probably hear it still. But again, a great lesson. It was one of the most toe-curlingly embarrassing moments of my broadcasting career but I just had to pick myself up, laugh it off and carry on broadcasting. As one of my old bosses used to reassuringly say, 'It's not life and death, it's only rock and roll'. This of course doesn't apply as good advice if you decide to go into medicine!

* * *

I will always love the radio most as that's where I started out and it's where I feel as a broadcaster you can be most honest, speaking from the heart without having to worry about what your face, body and hands are doing. Though this was before the advent of high-definition cameras on the radio. I mean, what a ridiculous idea. I understand in the current modern era that they provide a source of handy clips for social-media content, but I couldn't scratch my nose, roll my eyes or wear some dodgy clothes without getting a load of texts and Twitter messages from watchful listeners glued to the live feed!

So, I thought, 'in for a penny in for a pound' and after a few years freelancing at various London stations, including LBC, BBC London and BBC 5 Live, I decided the time was right to push into a bit of TV work to try something new. As the shy girl this was something that thrilled and terrified me in equal measure, but I have always been of the opinion that in life you need to challenge yourself and try out the things that scare you. I think this particularly applies to your twenties and thirties, which are the best times for testing new waters while blinded by the innocence of youth.

I fancied myself as a bit of a sports fan. Unlike your daddy, I've never massively been into football. I think it's because I'm Welsh, and in Wales we like rugby! But I loved watching all other sports – Formula 1, athletics, showjumping, three-day eventing, swimming. I saw it as my natural niche. A bit of asking in the right places got me some shifts reading the sports news on the BBC News Channel and I threw myself into it with all I had. Unfortunately, I found out the world of TV can be a tough one. I made the mistake of going in thinking I'd jazz up the dress code a bit; I now cringe when I see screen-grabs of the awful clothes and jewellery I used to wear. But you've got to try things out to know whether they work for you or not. I found out that fussy clothes do not! Most of the sports team were lovely to me, but I think the odd one thought I didn't know my sports well enough and made it not such a fun place to work. I cursed these chauvinists under my breath and moved on because you can't waste too much time on people who don't get you.

The then boss of the BBC News Channel seemed to believe in me though and I got my first stab at being a network rolling newsreader. It was a hugely exciting time and while suffering with imposter syndrome for much of it, feeling like I wasn't good enough and that someone would find me out, I thoroughly enjoyed every shift. If I tell you the shifts ran on air from midnight to 5 a.m. you'll understand that to stay awake during those hours I must really have loved it.

For a news junkie it is hard to compare anything to the excitement of breaking news as it is happening and being kept on your toes throughout. I guess it's a little like the buzz a rock star would get from being on stage, but with less leather, booze and singing, and no line of sight to your audience members!

I broke the news of some major stories during that time including the harrowing Norway attacks of 2011 when a lone-wolf terrorist called Anders Behring Breivik killed seventy-seven people in a car-bomb attack in Oslo and a mass shooting on Utøya Island where a children's summer camp was being held. It was difficult to piece the news together as snippets of information came through all afternoon. As my co-presenter and I spoke to more witnesses and members of the emergency services on the ground in Norway, the awful picture of what had taken place began to become clearer. Sometimes as a presenter you have to deal with harrowing details of stories with a slight detachment to maintain an air of professionalism. But always I tried to speak to guests with as much empathy and compassion as I could.

One very difficult night for me, as far as breaking news goes, came on the radio. I was the late newsreader on BBC 5 Live back in 2008 as news of the Mumbai terror attacks began to filter through. As it was a big sports night I was the main news voice at the station and was dispatched to the studio to present rolling coverage as more details came in. There was no running order really, as the producers were working hard to find eyewitnesses and I'd get a quick shout in my headphones about who I was about to speak to and would just get on with trying to find out what was happening. One man that I spoke to was actually in one of the hotels that was under siege. He said he was talking to us from the ballroom of the hotel where he was hiding with a number of other guests. He sounded so calm and collected when I spoke with him. My last words to him were that I hoped he would stay safe and get out of there soon. But he didn't. I arrived for my shift the next night to be told he was one of the people who'd been killed. I was numb as I processed that piece of information. Then, as I sat at the news desk to read through the 7 p.m. bulletin, I realized that his death was referenced in one of the news stories and I would have to keep repeating it all night. I broke down in tears as I just felt I couldn't do it. It was too close to home after having been one of the last people that he spoke to. One of our usually stern bosses kindly suggested I take the night off and escorted me back to the car park as the tears poured down my face. You can't always keep up that solid air of professionalism. Broadcasters are only human and sometimes dealing with these awful events can break us a little bit. But Fred, as always in the situations when you need to have your moment out, cry your tears for the people affected by these terrible atrocities then get back to doing the job, whatever that may be for you.

Another tragic night of news on a different level was the time in early 2012 when the death of legendary songstress Whitney Houston became known about two minutes before our first BBC World bulletin at 1 a.m. I was the first UK newsreader to break the news of her death. We rolled with the details of her untimely passing throughout the early hours of the morning. I was quite a fan of Whitney in the eighties – and you have to understand that as a journalist, even tragic stories like this carry with them an air of excitement as you piece together what's happened. It was a subject I knew a lot about and it actually made a night of being kept on my toes with last-minute interviewees one where, by the end of the shift – and this is something that happens so frequently – there was a point at which the sadness at the news almost turned into a privilege and pleasure when looking back on an icon's amazing career.

Talking of privilege, I had the honour and privilege to work alongside some brilliant broadcasters in my time at BBC 5 Live, chief among them the mercurial Richard Bacon. His late show which ran from 10 p.m. to 1 a.m. Monday to Thursday was the first regular show on which I read the news on 5 Live. I would sit in the studio for the full three hours, and as well as reading the news, I would also keep an eye on the texts that listeners were sending in and chip in on any of the more chatty moments with guests. It was one of the most fun shows I have worked on.

Richard had an eclectic mix of friends and contacts who would sit in the studio with us as 'presenter's friends' and because it is late-night radio, there is much more scope for ripping up the traditional news-show running order and having a bit of fun. And you know Mummy loves fun, Freddie! Towards the end of the show we'd all start to flag a bit, as 1 a.m. is a pretty late finish. And Richard in particular said he needed something to keep his focus during the last half an hour of the show. He's since been diagnosed with ADHD, something he has talked openly about, which really explains why the closing section of his show proved more of a challenge. And so the Special Half Hour was born. You only knew about the Special Half Hour if you were listening and happened to catch the strains of the 'William Tell Overture' that introduced it at 12.30 a.m. Rich joked that other listeners were lazy and missing out on what we began to refer to as the SHH. We would never reference it in any other part of the show and any guests that did were blackballed by the SHH members.

Among a certain group of 5 Live listeners TV presenter Nick Knowles's name is still mud after he mentioned the SHH at 10.45 one night. Did he not know the rules?! It was one of the most interactive and brilliant pieces of radio I've ever had the pleasure to be a part of. I'm really breaking the rules by talking about it, but I think the members of the SHH will forgive me this one time, Freddie. They set up a Facebook group – with 11,000 members at its peak – where they would post suggestions for games to play and topics to talk about. Discussions included, 'Why do cats not walk on tin foil?' We had games like SHH Cluedo, where listeners would tell us their name, where they were listening right at that moment and what object was closest to their left. And they weren't afraid to pull Richard up if they didn't like the content he was creating, 'Temporary Celebrity Friend' never went the distance. We even had pin badges that read 'SHH' that listeners could get if they had some great input into the show. I still get messages now asking if I have any more to send out!

We held the SHH's first birthday party in Richard's house in London, where his kitchen and lounge were packed with the most loyal SHHers and various celebrities, including TV and radio presenter Chris Evans and philosopher Alain de Botton – I told you he had eclectic friends! It was such a fun night. Eventually, when the time came for Richard to move on up to the 5 Live afternoon show, we even held a Special Half Hour funeral at a packed BBC Radio Theatre in Broadcasting House in central London. The stalls were packed with listeners and this one time we gave the SHH the full hour of radio time it deserved. Richard and I sat on the stage, both wearing black. I even bought a black funeral veil for the occasion – I took the SHH seriously! We sat on the stage with our funeral running orders in hand, me holding a white rose that one of the listeners had dashed down to hand to me. There was a sermon, a reading of W. H. Auden's 'Stop All the Clocks' and a rousing rendition of 'Jerusalem'. It was a fitting send-off for a fabulous bit of radio. I'm still in contact with many of the most active SHH contributors who actually became friends – Rita, Jon, Marc, Bri, Simon and the gang. We won an award in that same radio theatre a few months later – which I went to collect with Richard and Paul Bond, one of the producers – for the most creative piece of radio. The award is actually a slate from the roof of the original Broadcasting House and I hope is still on the mantelpiece. My involvement in that funny little half hour just as I started my career with BBC 5 Live is one of the bits I'm most proud of and most enjoyed.

Another fun appearance that came about thanks to Richard Bacon was my most talked-about TV appearance. You can read all the TV news bulletins you like and the majority of people will barely raise an eyebrow. Appear for about ten seconds on Armando Iannucci's cult political comedy *The Thick of It* and you get texts and messages from people years later when they catch the repeat on TV! Armando (we're not really on first-name terms but I shook his hand and he was very nice) wrote one of the episodes around a radio appearance by two of the main characters – Nicola Murray played by Rebecca Front and Roger Allam performing the role of Peter Mannion. They go head-to-head on who else's show ... but Richard Bacon's of course. I played my role of newsreader with aplomb. I really don't think even an Oscar-winning actor could have done my 'open door ... walk into studio ... sit down ... put headphones on' moment any better. I even got a credit in the show titles which means I'm listed on the Internet Movie Database (IMDB) website as an actor! Rachael Hodges ... Herself. If there's one role I was born to play in this life it's myself. Also, in between takes Rebecca Front whispered to me that she liked my jacket which really was the high point of the whole day!

Through my work, which I always tell people never feels like a proper job as it's too fun, I've been lucky enough to attend some amazing events. We got to watch the Queen's Diamond Jubilee Concert in 2012 from our makeshift studio at the edge of The Mall. We were just metres away from the stand the Royal Family was sitting in, so could look down on the Queen, Prince William et al. We may or may not have gone down there after the concert to take pictures in their seats and I also may or may not have Princess Anne's laminated reserved-seat sign knocking about somewhere at home. A bit of close-up royal watching was almost more fascinating than the amazing concert that was put on, featuring Take That, Elton John and Paul McCartney among others. There was also the most incredible light show projected onto the front of Buckingham Palace. By this time I was working on the late-night show with the brilliant Tony Livesey, who's another presenter I had a huge amount of fun working with and now get the pleasure of presenting BBC 5 Live *Drive* with him every Friday. I would again sit in studio, by this time up in MediaCityUK in Manchester, and it was during that show I had my top moment of hysteria on the airwaves. It involved trying to read out a list of famous 'Randys', and a texter told us there was a US politician by the name of 'Randy Bumgardener'. Well, it made me chuckle when I first read it off air and when I came to try and say it on air I just couldn't get the name out! Cue a lot of Tony in his Burnley accent asking 'Randy WHO??' as I sat in silent fits of giggles with tears pouring down my face. If I hear it back now I will still end up crying with laughter. Those late-night radio days were good times.

It was with Tony again that we headed to an outside broadcast at Silverstone at the start of the Formula 1 Grand Prix weekend. At the time I was hugely into F1 and couldn't wait for the programme which had loads of my favourite motor-racing guests ready to chat. We were based at a very busy White Horse pub in Silverstone village. I'd been lucky enough to go and pre-record a segment for the show with Paul Hawkins, the programme's sports reader, at an F1 simulator used by many of the younger drivers to practise in. We were given tips by a driver called Max Chilton, who at the time was still a rookie but who eventually made the move up to F1. Mummy is an excellent driver, Freddie – it's something I pride myself on. I once got an award left on my car for my top reverse parking. And I made sure I beat Paul around that simulator course! See, who can really call that work? It was so much fun. So we all arrived in Silverstone in the early afternoon ready for a fun-packed motor-racing extravaganza ... just as the news broke that the Sunday tabloid newspaper the *News of the World* was to close in the wake of the phone-hacking scandal. Running orders were ripped up, teeth gnashed and many guests on the programme were rearranged to talk about what was a pretty historic event. That is the nature of live broadcasting and working in news – sometimes the best-laid plans have to change. But they still played the audio of me beating Paul in the race in the F1 simulator, so it wasn't an entirely wasted trip!

After I moved north with the BBC in 2011, on my path of destiny to meet your dad, it became increasingly difficult to get back down to London for overnight TV shifts on a weekend when working full-time. And I had better things to do, now I had the love of my life to hang out with. But my short tenure as a network newsreader will remain one of the most exhilarating times of my life workwise. I still carried on with a bit of local TV when I arrived in the north, co-presenting the main evening show from time to time. And I presented the regional breakfast bulletins while I was pregnant with you – right up to thirty-seven weeks. It was kind of your first TV appearance, though the camera shot was mainly head and shoulders. I had the enormous fluid-retaining face but the viewers couldn't see the bump to make sense of it – I think a lot of them just thought I'd put on weight!

So, I guess my advice here, with the move from London to Cheshire, is to grab the opportunities when they come along and make the most of them, but never worry when the time comes to move on to the next big thing in your life, whatever that may be.

Chapter 4

I ABSOLUTELY DO

This seems a good point to go back to when I met Daddy. After the ski holiday with the new 'cheese fat allowing' trousers, we had the most amazing first year getting to know each other. It was 2012, the year of the London Olympics, and for us it was just a wonderful time to be alive. Our relationship moved at a quick but reasonable pace, just quick enough not to elicit any raised eyebrows at the speed of our romance. As I've already mentioned I knew from the moment I met Daddy (the one I remembered at least) that I would marry this man. I think he caught up a couple of months later!

That first year, after our first kiss in January, we skied in St Anton in March and went on to have wonderful dancing fun – tie on head (Daddy), bright-eyed clapping and grinning (Mummy) – at good friends' weddings through the summer. We met and got to know each other's families and by the end of the summer we had decided to get a dog and move in together. I had grown up with golden retrievers as family pets but Daddy, though coming from two farming families, had never lived with a dog in the house. We tossed around the idea like you do and, in the end, it was Daddy who really pushed for having a dog while I reminded him it was going to be a big responsibility! But oh my, it was the best thing we ever did getting our first dog and your best pal, Bodie. He has been such a shining beacon of joy through our time with him and I hope you still have fond memories of him too. More on our love affair with Bodie later. Let's get back to me and your dad.

When we decided to buy Bodie, I was still living in my flat in Hale with your dad down the road. So, we started the process of finding a rental property together and of course I got my heart set on a fairly pricey three-bed in Alderley Edge. It was probably a touch above our budget but sometimes you've just got to go with what makes you happy. And I was so happy in that house. It was where we fell more deeply in love, planned our wedding and you together, and I have always looked back on it as one of the happiest times. I loved to stroll down the high street in Alderley checking out the WAGS' clothes, while your dad was always overjoyed to bump into some ex-footballer or other outside Waitrose and get to chat to them through the medium of Bodie – dogs are such great ice-breakers.

I had spent most of that year gripped by Olympic fever, as this was a once-in-a-lifetime event in the UK and I spent hours trawling the London 2012 ticketing website for access to all sorts of events from rowing to volleyball to athletics. The very high point of my ticket-buying skills came when I managed to snag a pair of tickets for the Men's 100m Final at the Olympic Stadium. Your dad and I went and watched Usain Bolt light up the track with gold. I've always been a huge fan of any kind of big sporting event, I love that feeling of unity and joint elation among sports fans. Joy that can be shared among many is always exponential. But I know you will learn this from Daddy: every time my back is turned that TV changes from whatever mindless reality show I'm watching to any kind of sport or sports news! There will just be no escaping it. Though you are currently the 'troll-tyrant', always in charge of the controller and demanding the TV is changed onto *Octonauts*, *Peter Rabbit* or *Carl the Super-Truck*. They say the one who controls the TV holds the power, so make of that what you will!

A few weeks after the London Olympics drew to a close in a Britpop extravaganza that included the Spice Girls, George Michael and the Pet Shop Boys, we headed off to Los Angeles on what will always be one of my favourite holidays. It was a fairly last-minute decision to go and as ever one we probably couldn't afford but, in my experience, those are always the best kind of trips and nights out, unplanned and low on expectation.

We flew off from Manchester to LA via Chicago to stay with one of your dad's best friends, Chris Whittle – or Uncle Captain as he's more commonly known – who was one of the most generous hosts I have ever known. He not only gave up his bedroom for us for the duration of our stay in his one-bed flat, but also proceeded to give us the best insider tour of the City of Angels ever. At the time Uncle Captain was working as a paparazzi photographer (he is the politest and least pushy example of this you would ever find) and some of our tour time was taken up with stalking celebrities on street corners, which for your gossip-mag-loving mummy was an absolute thrill! All this in beautiful sunshine and among the gorgeous, stylish little shops of LA – I was smitten. One of my small regrets in life is never having spent any time living abroad and I always said after this trip that LA would have been the place for me had I decided to fly the UK nest.

We spent one particularly happy afternoon stalking actor-turned-politician Arnold Schwarzenegger after Uncle Captain spotted his enormous monster truck of a vehicle parked outside his offices.

We were not the only ones to have noticed this showy vehicle and one slightly inebriated couple decided to hold a full-blown photo shoot with the girlfriend hanging from the bull bars on the front! Luckily, they had staggered off by the time the Terminator strolled out in his smart office attire or who knows what could have happened. Sometimes the showiest cars and possessions can really attract the wrong kind of attention. Often understated shows way more class.

The rest of our trip involved riding bikes down Venice Beach while looking out for the singer-songwriter, Pink. Spotting the celebs' houses in Malibu, they looked pretty unassuming from the road but all faced out onto a magical view of the ocean – real 'don't judge a book by its cover' territory and a reminder to 'always think what the view is like from the other side'. Uncle Captain skilfully navigated us around the gazillion-lane highways of LA that are certainly NOT meant for tourists in hire cars. I got to hold up shopping bags on Rodeo Drive outside the shop where Julia Roberts had her own 'don't judge a book' moment in *Pretty Woman* – 'You work on commission, right? Big mistake. Big. Huge. I have to go shopping now!' – which is still my favourite snobbery slap-down ever. And I'll let Daddy fill you in on the day he ate a breakfast burrito that according to the menu contained 2,000 calories. He didn't eat again for a good two days.

We came back from LA, took delivery of puppy Bodie the very next day and settled into our life as a three in Alderley Edge. We spent Christmas there with Grandma and Grandad Hodges, with Daddy doing his usual spectacular job of cooking the turkey. I hope you inherit his kitchen skills and not mine as I am still ashamed to say that while I love eating it, I hate cooking food and have been known to mess up boiling an egg (they will explode if you leave them in the saucepan too long).

Then came our next ski trip to Méribel in France and right around this time I started to get an inkling that things were progressing on to the next stage of our relationship – engagement and marriage. I mostly deduced this when one day Daddy handed me his iPad to look at something and I spotted the other open tabs were all links to jewellers and engagement rings! I did an admirable job of internalizing my squeals of excitement of course and pretended I'd seen nothing. There is a lot of artifice involved in the ritual of getting engaged and one must respect the process. Or so I thought …

Knowing he was looking at rings and that there was a ski holiday coming up, I put two and two together and was highly expectant of a proposal on the French slopes. As it turned out, so did my poor father, your grandad, who Daddy had FaceTimed just before to ask if he would be happy for us to marry. He was of course overjoyed! But he was also confused by the timing. Daddy had decided not to take the expensive ring he had bought for me abroad and instead to pop the question when we got home. I wondered why your normally 'message-lite' grandad suddenly turned into a bit of a holiday stalker with constant text messages every day asking me how the trip was going! And then, to my embarrassment, I even argued with Daddy as the expected proposal never came. I was upset to think I had thought he wanted to get married soon but I'd got it so wrong. I arrived home from Méribel on the Sunday night in a bit of a two-day funk. You see, when I get in a mood, I find it VERY difficult to get out of it. And so far, Freddie, you are just the same! When something upsets us, it can take hours for us to come down off our grumpy high horses. Nothing anyone can say or do will make the mood lift any quicker but suddenly something will snap us out of it and all will be well with the world again. For you right now it is Fireman Sam. For me that day it was a diamond ring.

And this is how our engagement story came to be one where we were dressed in onesies. These giant, baggy, adult romper suits were quite in-fashion leisurewear back then and your dad and I had, by complete coincidence, bought each other 'his and hers' versions for Christmas. We had thrown them on when we got back from the airport and I was still in my 'he doesn't want to marry me' mood. Daddy began to ask if I wanted a present to cheer me up, and though I hate to make myself sound shallow, my ears pricked straight up! What sort of present? A shiny one?! Uh, yes please. Then he left me sitting downstairs on the sofa for over half an hour wondering what on earth was going on.

As it turned out he was upstairs letting both our families know that 'Operation Engagement' was about to get into full swing. This came as welcome relief to poor Grandad Hodges, as both he and Grandma had been questioning his sanity over the previous week as to whether he had actually received a call from your daddy asking for my hand in marriage at all. My first inkling that this was the 'THIS IS IT MOMENT' is when he strode back into the room, resplendent in his navy onesie, and gave me a massive hug. I could feel his heart beating through his chest!

Then, he dropped onto one knee and pulled a beautifully polished wooden ring box out of his pocket. Then my heart started beating out of my chest as I realized this was the moment. He opened the box and said, 'I was wondering if you would like to marry me.' I replied, 'Of course! I would love to!' My first thought on glancing at the ring was that it was too big to be real and must have been a 'fake placeholder' dress ring. But no, Daddy had done the best job of picking the most beautiful ring himself. My hints about loving emerald-cut diamonds had hit home. I love their sleek lines and simplicity. And clever Daddy had gone straight to the jewellery supplier to get more for his money.

It was set on diamond shoulders and I just could, not, stop, staring at it! I was like Gollum with his 'precious' and it really did snap me out of that mood! You don't always need extravagant gestures to cheer someone up, but sometimes only diamonds will do. That ring and my wedding ring we had made to match are yours, Freddie, to do with what you will, be it propose, save as a keepsake or just get out and laugh at how Mummy's first engagement pictures involved her wearing a onesie and no make-up.

Chapter 5

WHAT A WEDDING!

If the engagement pictures weren't good, then I was determined the wedding pictures would be the opposite, so I set about organizing the wedding of the century. I had always known I would get married and harboured some ideas of a big white affair, but had never wanted to think too deeply about it before it was actually happening. It's way more fun to come to these things with fresh eyes and enthusiasm. I was never one of those girls with a ring binder of wedding ideas they've kept since they were little, or perhaps that doesn't even happen and I've just watched too many of those cheesy movies we discussed earlier.

The proposal in the onesies took place in March 2013 and I knew that I wanted to get married asap so we could get a baby Freddie in our lives, as by this time I was approaching thirty-five, the age at which they start scaring women with alarm bells about declining chances of having a child. In my head September seemed like a good month, as often the weather in the summer months is disappointing and in April and September there seems to be more chance of staying dry. Luckily, when Daddy and I had the 'when shall we make this happen?' conversation that night, we both said 'September?' at the same moment. That gave us just under six months to turn it around. It may sound a lot to you now, but in wedding-planning terms that's the blink of an eye. Some venues are booked up years in advance, as are photographers, and it takes a few months if you want a bespoke dress (obviously Mummy did!). But I was more than up for the challenge. I got folders, highlighters, brochures and set about planning with the kind of enthusiasm only mustered by the newly engaged. I used to get laughed at by colleagues at work as I took my 'wedding-planning bag' with me everywhere to keep track of what I was booking.

First up, the tricky bit of setting the budget. Grandma and Grandad had very generously set aside way more of their retirement fund than I thought possible, and Gran and Grumpy also kindly contributed a very large amount and paid for the honeymoon. Plus, I kept chucking in any extra pay I had to justify my extra bits of spending. As you'll already have gathered, I think, I don't have the best budgeting skills and found it very difficult to make economies. It's so easy to get carried away in the 'more, more, more' culture of weddings and I am not ashamed to admit that I got swept up in the madness. In my opinion, I was only doing it once, I'd waited thirty-four years to do it and my God I was going to do it right!

We quickly nailed down the venue of my dreams. I wanted to get married near home back in South Wales, but there weren't many places around Cardiff that fitted the bill for me. Then, a bit like Brigadoon on a misty night, my perfect wedding venue magically emerged ... the beautiful, stunning Llangoed Hall, which was just forty-five minutes up the road from home but I had never known was there. A bit like Daddy, it was just waiting for me to find it. I don't know if it will still be the same if you were to visit it now, but back then it was just like having our own country house for the weekend. As soon as we approached it and I got my first peek of its beautiful Edwardian frontage through the trees I knew this was the place we would get married.

It was steeped in Welsh history and the oldest part of the building was believed to have been used to house the first Welsh parliament during the sixth century AD. Latterly it had been owned for a time by Sir Bernard Ashley, husband of the renowned Welsh fashion designer Laura Ashley, and one of the first aprons Laura had ever sewn is proudly framed and hung on one of the walls. History and heritage are so important to what makes us who we are and I guess this is why I'm writing all this down for you. I was born and brought up in Wales and even though I lost my accent after many years of newsreading I am still Welsh through and through. There have been a number of jovial arguments between your father and me about which side you'd play for should you take up rugby or football internationally! We eventually settled on you being an England and Wales cricketer to cover both sides – no pressure! I know that living in England and spending time watching sport with your dad that you'll be English first, but I hope you'll still have that Welsh dragon roaring inside you from your mummy.

Laura Ashley never lived at Llangoed Hall as she died in 1985, two years before her husband bought it. However, Sir Bernard spent many happy years there with his family and one of the lovely things about it was that their family pictures still stood on mantelpieces and hung on the walls. The hotel had just been bought by a new owner and a brand-new refurb was finished in time for our wedding. I couldn't have found a more perfect place to spend our wedding weekend. There was no reception and the staff emerged as if by magic, the team of Calum, Brian and co. seeming to know what drinks and food you needed before you did. Downstairs there was a billiard room, perfect for Daddy to have a late-night whiskey, an amazing sitting room for chilling out and reading and the gorgeous pale-blue dining room with its wonderful collection of artwork.

As you may gather, we totally fell in love with it and it's a love affair that has endured. Whenever we can we go back to celebrate special occasions and always stay in our wedding suite, Paulton's, a huge beautiful room decorated in pale blue that has a bigger floor space than most homes I've inhabited. We always call it our happy place, our home from home. We go back to familiar faces and scenes, and the happy dancing memories of our wedding party become vivid in the mind again. I do hope you will still get to visit there and love it in the years to come as we do.

A weekend was free that September and so the venue was settled, then next on the money-drain list was THE DRESS! I've always been someone who has fussed over their appearance, with hindsight way too much. But if you're ever going to look your best your wedding day is the day to do it on, isn't it? I had pored over wedding magazines and looked at different dress silhouettes. I fancied full ballgown as I figured my wedding day might be the only one where I got to wear something so extravagant. Wedding-dress shops are their very own breed, as unlike normal shops you can't just wander in uninvited and start trying things on off the rails. Appointments must be booked and strict entry criteria met.

I haphazardly booked two totally different appointments for the first (and what turned out to be the only) day of wedding-dress shopping. I set off with Grandma, Gran and your dad's sister, Auntie Claire, in tow. The two dress shops perfectly represented the old adage 'you get what you pay for', which I stand by to this day. The first was staffed by a suspicious lady who wouldn't give us clear prices on any of the dresses or tell us the designer or let us take pictures. I immediately knew when we stepped in there that none of the dresses would be 'the one'. So, I did what any self-respecting bride-to-be would do in that situation and set about using the appointment to try on the biggest most ridiculous dresses I could find in the shop to fall about laughing in! I did not feel bad after the woman practically chased us out of the door after trying to get me to put a deposit on a dress she had blatantly randomly priced to fit the budget I had suggested. The old cynic in me was well prepared for this kind of con, so I said thanks but no thanks and headed off to the next shop, which turned out to be the bridal shop of my dreams.

The bridal boutique Lace has long since closed down in Hale, but at the time it was like walking into a place where they'd read my mind about what I wanted in a dress. Helped by the lovely staff Katie and Lesley, I felt immediately at home. I could see the fabrics and styles of the dresses were exactly what I was looking for. Katie told me not to be swayed by a particular style of dress as things could be changed on all of them to make them bespoke. Now this sounded right up my alley, and as I noticed Grandma and Gran's faces getting a little tight at the prices I knew I was in the right spot! Katie had one of the designers she stocked in mind for me and what a perfect fit Caroline Castigliano and I were. I adore every one of her dresses, the material, the tailoring, the internal corsetry. Just perfect. I was lucky enough to wear a couple of her evening dresses in the following years and as soon as you put one near me I would instantly carry myself in a different way, courtesy of the magic dress that pours elegance into you.

We settled on a couple to try: one ballgown silhouette I'd seen online and one long, more fitted lace number. We carried this precious cargo of silk and lace down to the fitting rooms downstairs, a wonderful plush area with GLITTER IN THE CARPET! Hello, I was in my element.

The lace dress was fabulous and made me feel amazing, but as soon as I got into the ballgown and started swooshing my skirt around like a Disney princess then I knew that was the one. I've said it before, when you know, you know. Always try to tune in and trust your instincts whether you are buying a dress (you may prefer a suit but who knows!) or picking a life partner.

Of course, me being me, I couldn't have it just as it was. The bottom full-circle skirt was a duchess satin, with a corseted bodice and a light lace, three-quarter-sleeved, boat-necked top and low V at the back. (Your dad has just read this, snorting with laughter, saying all those details will mean nothing to you! But just in case you do appreciate the art of good dress construction I feel it is my legacy to leave these details behind …) It was all topped off with the signature Caroline Castigliano grey belt. But Mummy with her magpie tendencies had rather had her head turned by the amazing corded and beaded lace on the other dress that caught the light and sparkled as I moved. So, I had my own bespoke change made to the lace on top of the dress, a few extra hundred pounds added onto the bill and the deal was done! Deposits were paid and we headed off to drink some Prosecco to toast the most expensive clothing purchase I had ever made. Well, that your grandparents had ever made. After a Prosecco I persuaded Grandma not to discuss the finer details of dress finances with Grandad Hodges! This is not the last on the finished dress effect, as I ignore my own advice about instincts for a while, but we'll come back to the story of two veils later.

I should point out that while I may sound a bit like I'm coming across as a bridezilla here – even Katie from the bridal shop affectionately referred to me as 'her zilla' – I'm just a bit of a stickler for detail. I've always had the bad habit of procrastination, leaving stuff like exam revision until the last minute, but once I get started on a task

I like to do it with 100 per cent of my enthusiasm. Always remember that's all you can do, literally. Your dad climbs the walls every time a sportsperson says they 'gave it 110 per cent' because ... you can't! So, I didn't spend the whole budget on dresses and diamonds for me. Your dad has always loved his watches and I desperately wanted to buy him a super-swanky Breitling, which I absolutely loved. I got a blingy ring and Daddy got a blingy Breitling. By the time I'd paid it off about three years later, the battery had run out, you'd arrived and we couldn't afford the replacement battery, so the watch languished in a drawer unworn for a couple of years! In another piece of 'do as we say, not as we do' advice, it's much better to keep on top of this kind of life admin, get things fixed up asap and 'never leave a Breitling in the corner'! That, by the way, is a reference to another of Mummy's dodgy films, *Dirty Dancing*, which I hope is still a cult classic.

Venue and dress, photographer and cake nailed down, I then got all the other details sorted. The flower budget was a slight tension point between me and Daddy. Hell, let's face it, all my money-making decisions were! I wanted a lot of roses and larger-headed flowers set together in bouquets, obviously one of the most expensive ways of doing it. Flowers can add so much to a wedding but my gosh they are expensive. I found the perfect flower shop, Love Lily in Abergavenny, just up the road from Llangoed Hall. They produced my vision of peach, yellow, pinky blooms for the bouquets and table centrepieces better than I could ever have hoped. I still think in the photos they look good enough to eat.

I agreed to compromise budget-wise by decorating the church with flowers ourselves. This was definitely a job that Gran and her green-fingered skills had to be in charge of. And the church – I haven't even mentioned it yet!

As we were not technically of the parish we were getting married in, we had to meet the vicar, Reverend Charlesworth, henceforth referred to as Rev C! If I'd had any worries about getting married by a stranger, they were soon forgotten when I met this larger-than-life man of personality and stature, with his booming, resonant voice and cheeky sense of humour. He was such an integral part of the wedding. There were two churches in the parish that could accommodate our large number of guests. Llanstephan was a more ornate church up on a hill, which I was immediately put off because there was no concrete path and I had visions of my wedding shoes sinking into the mud!

But as we approached St Matthew's in the parish of Llandefalle, much like that first viewing of Llangoed Hall, a sense of magic set in. It was a snowy day in Wales and we glimpsed its rustic whitewashed walls though the black branches of the early spring trees that had yet to bud and we knew it was perfect. Huge and airy (and very cold!) inside, we pushed open the door and went in to explore. Built in the fifteenth century, it is simple and plain inside but with a beautiful fourteenth-century carved wooden screen that sits in front of the choir seats. Daddy and I had a little practice staying at the altar together and walking down the aisle. It gave us goosebumps and giggles in equal measure and we couldn't wait to do it for real a few months down the line.

And so, the wedding day flew around and I started the bridal process of pre-beautifying. I had done a lot of changing my mind over who should do my hair and make-up but all was now in place. I saw my trusted hairdresser, Leah, for my final colour and blow dry, tick one. I had beautiful lash extensions put on to pretty up my eyes, tick two. Gel nail varnish was applied in a salon in Alderley Edge, a soft pearlescent baby pink, tick three. Ah I was going to look so perfect … then I almost buggered it right up by doing something which in hindsight was unfathomably stupid! Hair removal is always a big thing for women and I'd previously had a process called threading done on my eyebrows, where they basically use two bits of cotton to pluck out the hairs. It is literally THE most painful beauty process I've ever experienced, but the results are worth the ten minutes of tears streaming down your face that you have to endure. Now all the bridal magazines – remember I had read THEM ALL – tell you not to make any drastic changes to your beauty routine in the lead-up to the big day. I had read this. Comprehended and understood. So, it must have been in a moment of pre-wedding insanity that I decided to go and get my WHOLE FACE threaded ... yep, that searing pain from forehead to jawline. I'm relatively fair-skinned, just like you, and I barely even have any noticeable facial hair and what I do have is obviously there for a reason. But I must have been harbouring some ideas of looking super-smooth in the close-up wedding shots.

Once the painful process was over the beautician, in her wisdom, decided not to put any cooling cream on my face afterwards in case it encouraged spots. So off I trotted back home to Daddy with my face as smooth as a new baby's bottom. By the time I arrived, that face was starting to get a little hot, then I caught sight of my cheeks in the reflection of the oven door and literally screamed. Turns out my skin is a bit sensitive and large sections of my face were coming out in bumpy areas of folliculitis! I still look back now and cringe at what an idiot I was. This was two days before the wedding and there was just no consoling me. Daddy tried his best – 'You can hardly tell ...' – as did Auntie Claire, but when the girls took a shocked intake of breath as I positioned myself in some good lighting while collecting my dress, I knew this was bad! Thankfully my GP cousin, your Uncle Robbie, came to the rescue with some quick-working antibiotics and lashings of aloe vera gel, so that come the wedding morning you could barely see it. Or that's what they all told me anyway! It remains one of my stupidest-ever decisions and I guess you can learn from that, my darling, even if the scenario is different, that if everything around you is going a bit crazy, try and keep a cool head and THINK about the outcomes of the decisions you're making.

I guess this also applies to the previously mentioned 'two veils'. In a magazine I spotted a lace-edged veil that looked so glamorous and fabulous that I decided it would be perfect with my dress. I had one made with matching lace by Caroline Castigliano that cost almost a THOUSAND POUNDS – I admit I had lost all sense of budget at this point – but when I came to try it on with the dress just a couple of weeks before the big day, something nagged at me. The lace of the veil across the lace sleeve of my dress was too much. Sometimes you've just got to bite the bullet, so I called Katie, ordered a plain, simple, long veil from Caroline and boxed up my expensive mishap, to be sold at a great loss via a wedding website, but hopefully to a bride who felt a million dollars in it.

* * *

I awoke on our wedding morning super-excited, after that first quick dash to the mirror to check on my skin. Auntie Claire, who was chief bridesmaid, was first to my room and the lady doing make-up and hair was due to arrive at 6.30 a.m. She actually got stuck in traffic at that time of day and was late arriving, and this is where my perfectly planned timings began to slide somewhat. We had the perfect bridal prep morning though. My old friends Auntie Jo and Auntie Rachael, who were my other bridesmaids, soon arrived and we set about turning that gorgeous suite with its four-poster bed into an absolute tip! We had a beautiful Llangoed Hall breakfast of salmon and scrambled eggs brought to the room and drank a couple of the obligatory glasses of Buck's Fizz. The make-up and hair lady slowly worked her way through all of us, though with hindsight she had perhaps taken on too many jobs to do solo. Suddenly I was aware the wedding planner at the hotel was getting antsy! But I was not to be rushed, there's a lot of stuff to put on in a wedding outfit. The details … I wore Grandma's garter on my leg which she had worn at her wedding to Grandad Hodges in 1967, that was my something old. The dress was obviously my something new. My borrowed was a beautiful set of pearl-and-diamond earrings and a pearl-and-diamond bracelet that were worth a fortune and had been kindly lent to me by a jewellery company called Green+Benz who I'd been introduced to through the bridal shop. I had found the most beautiful blue-and-white china-pattern pointy stiletto shoes from LK Bennett which I totally adored – my something blue. The look was topped off with a pearl-and-stone headpiece and all that remained was to attach my new light and perfect veil in place and I was good to go! But therein we had made another little mistake …

But first, this was the moment when I was almost overcome with emotion. I was dressed, feeling beautiful and all the planning and hard work was behind me. I was ready to go and marry the man of my dreams and enjoy our wedding day! Everyone else was at the church and as I walked carefully down the steps to meet Grandad, my eyes filled with tears. Now, like every self-respecting bride, I blinked these back so as not to ruin my make-up. Your Grandad Hodges was a man of few true heartfelt words – he was more likely to crack a one-liner! – but we had some lovely moments together stood in the hallway at Llangoed Hall, both ready for the biggest job of our lives.

So, we chatted and we waited for the car to return. Grandma and the bridesmaids had all been whisked off to the church in the vintage Daimler we had hired for the occasion. Now looking back this was not our best-ever decision, considering that the bridal party was a good twenty minutes late getting ready and the speed a vintage Daimler takes to do the five-mile round trip to the church and back can only be described as tediously slow. And so it came to pass that I will forever in the minds of our 160 or so guests be the LATEST BRIDAL ARRIVAL EVER. It was around forty minutes, I think. Remember I told you the church was old and rustic and cold? It also had no toilet. It still gives me a shiver down the spine to think of any poor souls who turned up early needing a wee then had to sit through forty minutes of 'is she coming?' then another hour of wedding!

It did at the very least give your dad a great ad-lib opener to his speech later about how one of the first things I told him about myself is that I hate it when people are late! I totally agree that this is ridiculous as your dad and I are never on time for anything. If we are the first to an event we literally spend the whole time voicing our shock. But generally, we are the latest. I believe the best advice is to try and aim to get to an event or meeting a good fifteen minutes before the stated time. We've just not quite managed that ourselves yet, so a challenge for you through life is to see if you can better our terrible tardy record and restore the good Bland name on the social scene!

* * *

Just the forty minutes late this time then, as I arrived at the church to the glorious sight of my beautiful best friends and bridesmaids in the flowing butter-yellow chiffon dresses. The weather was bright and dry so no big panic about my dress getting dirty on the floor – a major worry for me pre-wedding. Another example of my habit of blowing simple small concerns out of proportion, which I get from Grandma – it's on her side of the family! Always try not to worry about the things you cannot change.

It was time for a big, deep breath as the wonderful Rev C was waiting outside, sitting in a naturally formed seat in the stone wall of the perimeter of the church like the king of all he surveyed. He immediately put my stress and worry about keeping everyone waiting to one side with the simple phrase, 'The wedding never starts until the bride arrives', and then we formed into our bridal party and off we went down the stone path and to the doors of the church.

Honouring those Welsh roots of mine, we had booked a Welsh male voice choir to sing before and during the service, and what a wonderful sound they made. I will come on to my love of music later, but it's something I hope you will have too. The music was carefully chosen and I walked down the aisle on the arm of my dear daddy to the rich sound of the choir singing my favourite Welsh hymn, 'Calon Lân' – you may know by now it's an old perennial sung by Welsh rugby crowds at every game and is also the song my Welsh girls and I used to sing at the tops of our voices during taxi rides on nights out in our youth!

Just the thought of hearing it on that day now brings me out in goosebumps, as it is a beautiful song:

> Calon lân yn llawn daioni,
> Tecach yw na'r lili dlos:
> Dim ond calon lân all ganu
> Canu'r dydd a chanu'r nos.

This roughly translates as:

> A pure heart full of goodness
> Is fairer than the pretty lily,
> None but a pure heart can sing,
> Sing in the day and sing in the night.
> All about the Welsh love of singing!

The church was packed with all our closest friends and family, and I began to relax a little as I saw their smiling faces. No one looked too angry about my dreadfully late arrival (they'd save all their jokes for later) and I locked eyes with your daddy and dashed down the aisle at such a pace that Grandad had to tell me to slow down.

I arrived at the altar to stand next to Daddy and of course Rev C opened with a joke about me being late – I really just live to set up the jokes for other people to bat out of the park! And that set the tone for the service, which was one of great joy, laughter, serious moments and tears. I held myself together during the vows, doing my best to speak up in a loud and clear voice, keeping up my broadcasting credentials. It was your daddy whose voice broke during the vows, which I loved as it obviously meant so much to him. Unless he was choked up at picking a wife who would make him later for things than he already was!

The hymns were 'Love Divine, All Loves Excelling', which then always made me cry at future weddings because it was the last time I sung it with my daddy by my side before he died the following year. 'Lord of All Hopefulness', which I had loved since school, and of course, 'Cwm Rhondda' – 'Bread of Heaven', the hymn no Welsh wedding is complete without! Having the male voice choir leading the singing meant there was a rousing sound in the church. So often people are embarrassed to sing loudly at weddings, but take a note out of your Grandad Hodges' book on this one and sing as loud and proud as you can, even if you're not hitting the right notes! It's all about what you give it.

My friend Tracy read all of my favourite children's book, *Guess How Much I Love You*. In case you've forgotten, the answer is 'To the moon … and back', a sign-off I always use with your grandma on messages. Uncle Mark did an excellent job of a slightly saucy religious reading from the words of Solomon – he mostly kept a straight face which I'm sure you'll know by now is about as good as you can hope for from him!

Once the vows were exchanged we signed the register as the choir sung a Welsh hymn called 'Rachie', which was perfect as it's the shortened version of my name that all my close friends and family use. And of course, especially for your Liverpool-loving dad, a spine-tingling rendition of 'You'll Never Walk Alone' followed. We processed out of the church and the sunshine broke through the clouds at just that moment. It felt like someone was smiling down on us as we hugged friends and family at that little white church on the top of the hill with beautiful views across the sunny Wye Valley behind us.

Photos were taken and there was a small incident with a bracelet. We never quite got to the bottom of it and it was probably a little my fault. I had artfully stuffed the lovely dried-flower petal confetti I had ordered into little gauze bags, intending for people to pour it out into their hands to throw. But most chose, understandably, to go with a 'flinging from the bag' kind of action. Someone must have had an overarm action to rival Shane Warne because as well as flinging the confetti, a chunky pearl bracelet joined the shower of petals and made direct contact with the back window of the photographer's car, shattering it instantly! Being a typically oblivious bride, I had no idea this had happened until Steve, one of the best men, held up the offending bangle during the speeches later. We never did find out who the lady guest with the top bowling action was.

We headed back to Llangoed Hall in the Daimler, now a little behind schedule for our wedding breakfast timings. There seemed to have been a lot of pictures to take, and I was feeling the pressure to move the schedule along a bit under the stern gaze of the hotel wedding planner! I've always hated having my photo taken, as I'm always so hypercritical of how I look and too self-conscious to pull off a good pose. But I always wish I had more photos after I have been to places – it's a difficult trade-off. You want a record of precious moments, but you always want to live in them too. Always try and be present in what you're doing, take it in, make plenty of mental memories. And if there's time, get some Insta-worthy shots too!

I was, by the end of the photo-taking, to put it politely, a little grumpy. I kept having the glasses of our carefully chosen Prosecco and raspberry bellinis snatched from my hands to be whisked off to another location to pose in, looking wistfully into the distance. As we were walking through the rose garden for the umpteenth time and I was moaning at Daddy, he joked that we were nearly there and I should paste on a smile. I looked back and gave him an ironic rictus grin and that was the photo the photographer chose as her favourite! It just goes to show that even though a picture can show a thousand words, some of them may be unprintable …

After drinks and canapés on the croquet lawn, we headed into the wedding-breakfast room, which looked just as I'd dreamed. Llangoed Hall didn't go halves on the place settings. All top-notch crockery, silver cutlery and crystal glasses – I had a few concerns about how they might fare later with some of our more inebriated guests. All the beautiful pink, peach, yellow and cream flower accents were there with a garland across the top table and a mix of tall candelabra and low cake-stand centrepieces. The gazillion pounds I'd spent on beautiful bespoke menus and place settings was totally worth it. I'd agonized over whether to spend so much, but the thick, cream, luxurious card with golden writing set everything off perfectly. My good friend Uma described it as 'the classiest wedding set-up ever', which is the one comment I now use to totally justify the expense!

After beautiful food came the speeches. First up your grandad Hodges, who three months previously had had a massive operation to treat oesophageal cancer and was a shadow of his former self.

All my life I'd wondered what kind of speech he would give at my wedding, because as I said earlier, he was always prone to jokes not sentiment! He had been pretty wiped out in the lead-up to the wedding and your Grandma said she'd help with his speech. When I asked what they had so far, the answer was 'Well, we're going to say you like shoes ...'

So, never one to relinquish control, I thought it would be sensible for me to step in and give him a few subject areas to cover. I shouldn't have worried though because your grandad, 'Dave', rose to the occasion like a phoenix from the ashes. He had everyone in stitches and to a fresh crowd his old one-liners went down a storm! As I read in his eulogy at his funeral ten months later, one of our friends described it as 'the finest of father-of-the-bride speeches'.

Then came Daddy's turn. He kept himself manfully sober and I banned him from drinking red wine while sitting next to 'the dress'. He's likes a wild hand gesture and I had visions of him whacking a glass of red skywards and onto the perfect ivory dress mid-speech. So, he agreed to stay on the white, and for a man who loves his red wine that really was a gesture of true love. Daddy's speech was also a triumph – I think he missed his calling as a public speaker!

Steve and Will, the best men, followed with their two-man onslaught on Daddy's character. Along with the prop of that bracelet. Then we cleared the decks for the band to set up for the dancing. You can always judge the success of a wedding by the party and wow, what a party we had. I stayed firmly rooted to the dance floor for the night because I think if the bride is dancing then the guests have got to dance too. We had a brilliant live band that I'd spotted on a night out in Hale quite some time before we'd got engaged and had taken their details 'for a friend who was getting married soon', i.e. me!

Our first dance was to the top cheesy number, 'Can't Smile Without You' by King of Cheese, Barry Manilow. You know, I can't even remember now how it came to be 'our song'. But I remember many a car journey with your daddy when we were first together, when we would laughingly sing along to it together. Me in my best choirgirl voice and your daddy smiling at me, telling me how happy it made his heart to hear me sing. We'd been warned the hotel's sound system wasn't great with modern music and … disaster! Just as we began to sway along to the strains of old Bazza the sound system cut out! But this is why choosing a good cheesy number that everyone knows paid off because the encircled guests just carried on singing along, the band struck up and joined in, and what could have been a low point turned into one of my favourite moments of the day.

Daddy had a huge number of friends there as he's a popular guy and the one who caused all the issues with trying to trim down the guest list. And between them and my reprobate lot (I mean that affectionately, I have the most wonderful friends) it was an amazing night. I left the dance floor early on for a moment to take a breath alone in our suite and literally peel those lovely china-blue LK Bennett stilettos off my feet. The pain! I replaced them with a way more comfortable pair of white, chunky-heeled ankle boots. It meant the hem of my dress would drag on the floor (among many spilt drinks), but now the photos were done I didn't care. Which was good because I arrived back on the dance floor to a fully-fledged dance-off! Guests stood in a circle, clapping, while my friend Trace (who was a good few months pregnant at the time but can't resist a dance-off) pulled out a dance move that she calls 'the archer'. Your dad's best friend, Uncle Will, was ON ONE. After swooping up Rach my bridesmaid, and managing to pull half her dress down, his eyes locked on me like he sensed my fear! I was grabbed and whirled high into the air and I'm pretty sure the one rip in the lace of my dress (go and look at it and you'll find it in the middle of the front near the waist) was his handiwork. By some miracle he managed to plant me safely back on the floor and the night carried on.

I'm proud to say there was a human pyramid – with the all-important five-man base. And the top, top point of the night was when the band agreed to riff my favourite Killers song, 'Mr Brightside', even though it wasn't in their usual repertoire. There's an amazing video that I hope is still knocking about somewhere of the Killers fans among us in the crowd going wild, while other tipsy guests get jostled around the dance floor. I am front and centre, leaping up and down for all I'm worth, shouting the lyrics to your Auntie Jo and Tina and Janni at the top of my voice. It was a euphoric moment and a wonderful end to a wonderful day. I won't say it was as perfect as I had planned, for the many reasons listed above, but what a wonderful illustration of life. Life is never perfect my Fred, but it doesn't matter because as long as you don't dwell on the disappointing bits, another 'Mr Brightside' moment will be along before you know it.

Chapter 6

EXPANDING TEAM BLAND

There wasn't a moment to come down from the high of our wedding day as the next day we spent another lovely day with family at Llangoed Hall, dissecting the highs and lows of the wedding, before heading to Manchester Airport to enjoy a night in the luxury hotel, the Radisson Blu. Then it was off on honeymoon to the Maldives. I never thought I'd be a 'Maldives honeymoon' kind of girl, as I loftily thought it was a bit of a cliché, but when it came to poring over the travel brochures and looking at suggested itineraries for dashing around on safaris or city trips, the notion of just lazing on a beach after the wedding became more and more appealing!

And it was a perfect ten days, we really could not have wished for better. We picked a mid-range island – you can spend an almost infinite amount on some hotels there – and chose a beach bungalow rather than one over water so we could stay for longer. My feet didn't see a pair of shoes for the whole trip as you don't need them on the sandy paths and sand-floored bar and restaurant.

Daddy and I had such a wonderful time, enjoying romantic candle-lit dinners on the beach with expensive champagne. Strangely, the waiters all had an odd fascination with making leaves into insect shapes and presenting them to us like prizes. As I mentioned earlier, I'm not a huge fan of insects, so having a cricket or locust lobbed next to my plate of seafood every so often didn't actually enhance the atmosphere! They did make for excellent tipsy photo props though …

We snorkelled in the reef around the island and despite having learnt to dive years before, I had a full-on panic and leapt out of the water *Jaws*-style when I noticed three tiny reef sharks circling us. I think my bravery has waned somewhat as I've got older. We went on a sunset boat cruise and swam with a couple of huge and awe-inspiring whale sharks. We'd laze on the lovely white sofas around the island's infinity pool drinking Tom Collins cocktails and letting all of the wedding stresses go. Daddy taught me how to play chess and I became OBSESSED – have I mentioned my competitive side? I was desperate to beat him and played every night. In fact, our only cross word the whole time was when he suggested we didn't play one night. It didn't go down well with me, so the chessboard came out again and we played! I beat him once only, but what a golden moment that was.

But my absolute favourite part of the trip was the stars. On such a tiny island out in the Indian Ocean there is no light pollution to dim their beauty and every night, as we walked back along the star-lit beach after dinner, I would crane my neck to look at them. We'd often take a wander down the jetty and lay on our backs, listening to the waves gently pat the wooden slats while gazing up at those sparkling, dazzling lights. Nature is such a beautiful and wonderful thing, Freddie. When life and your mind get busy and it feels like too much, find your quiet spot, lay back and look up at those beautiful stars. Breathe in and breathe out and think of me, sparkling back down at you with every fibre of my being.

* * *

We arrived back from our honeymoon tanned, refreshed and even more in love and ready to add to Team Bland. The two of us and Bodie were a good start but we both desperately wanted a baby as soon as possible. Having not thought much about fertility through my twenties, I had become aware as soon as I'd met Daddy that perhaps the old biological clock was starting to tick a bit louder. And then, of course, my body decided to throw a spanner in the works. It turns out it is very good at growing things it shouldn't and I am not very good at noticing that. It's funny because I always thought I was hyper-aware of changes to my body. Having considered myself super-fit and healthy, always whizzing through those medical questionnaires you fill in with 'no history of anything dodgy', I was about to make my first foray into the world of hospital gowns and general anaesthetics.

In the lead-up to the wedding I'd been experiencing some quite sharp lower-tummy pains and was sent off for a scan by the doctor. I blithely skipped off to the scanning department expecting all to be fine and dandy. Just like with a pregnancy scan, cold gel was put on my tummy and chased around with the hand probe. When I cheerily asked the radiographer what she could see, expecting to hear 'It all looks normal', what I got was 'I can see quite a large mass actually' … I have now, post-cancer, become very used to hearing bad news and undergoing medical procedures, but at that time it came as quite the shock. I nearly fell off the bed and was too scared to ask any details. It turned out to be a cyst on one of my ovaries.

Here's the science bit and I'm sorry if you're now a teenager and trying to claw your own eyes out rather than read about fertility and babies! It's quite normal for a cyst to form after an egg has been released from an ovary each month, but they normally burst harmlessly and wither away. Well this one didn't, as my crazy body just kept on growing it until it was a good 12 cm – about the size of a grapefruit! I was almost impressed. My lovely gynaecologist, Mr Pickersgill (more of him later), expressed surprise that I hadn't noticed it there. I'd kind of just thought I was bloated or that the hard bit underneath my tummy was just abs – wishful thinking! Well, now it had been picked up the grapefruit couldn't stay, and this was only five weeks before the wedding day. Luckily Mr P was able to remove it through keyhole surgery that only involved three tiny cuts in my tummy. The recovery was quick, and I thought my hospital days were over.

So, off the back of that fertility scare Daddy and I were overjoyed to get a positive pregnancy test just a month after the wedding. We were almost smug in our happiness at how easy it was. Finding soulmate – done. Wedding of dreams – tick. Baby immediately on the way – easy. But that's not how life is unfortunately, my Fred, and sometimes things do not run smoothly. My initial elation at being pregnant soon turned to intense anxiety when I realized the medication I'd been taking for some time to stave off minor panic attacks was not allowed while pregnant. That of course sent me into an intense period of anxiety and I did not enjoy those first twelve weeks. A sense of foreboding overcame me, but I dragged myself through to the twelve-week scan, desperate to get out the other side and be able to explain some of my stranger and more stressy behaviour to friends and colleagues.

I lay back on the bed ready to exchange watery smiles with your dad over the happy images of the ultrasound. But as the radiographer began to look at the grainy images on the screen, clicking and taking measurements, the mood in the room turned suddenly cold. All looked fine with baby she said, apart from one measurement which was coming up very high. At the twelve-week scan they can measure an area of fluid at the back of a baby's neck – if it's too thick it can be a sign of abnormality. And this measurement was way above normal. I lay with silent tears dripping down the sides of my face and splashing onto the plastic bed. Daddy, not for the last time when bad news was delivered, started to ask if it was hot in the room. He had to remove his enormous woolly jumper and put his head between his knees as nurses fussed around him. We were sent to a 'bad news waiting room', which is never good. The consultant had reviewed the scans and the baby seemed to have a lot of issues. We were referred to the specialist Foetal Medicine Unit in Manchester for more tests and were told the baby had conditions called hydrops fetalis and cystic hygroma and had no chance of surviving to term. We had to make the heartbreaking decision to terminate the pregnancy. We were totally floored by the whole experience. For two people who take such joy in life and live to be happy, it was our first real experience of loss and true heartbreak.

With typically ironic timing, this all happened in the lead-up to Christmas, and so while everyone around us was sparkling in sequins and quaffing champagne and mince pies, I was sinking into a black hole of despair. It was also the last Christmas we had Grandad Hodges with us. He was not feeling great and we were about to find out his cancer was back. But I almost look back fondly on our time sat in companionable misery on the sofa of our house in Alderley Edge, eyeing each other knowingly, him in pain from the cancer, me in pain from the loss of my first baby. What a Scrooge-like pair we made.

They say time is a great healer, my Fred, and they are right. As the winter moved into spring and the days brightened, then so did my mood. But you, my little sausage, still evaded us. Every month we kept trying for that positive pregnancy test, knowing how easy it had been the first time, but every month … no pink lines. We even signed up at the IVF clinic thinking our chances were diminishing. We knew I still had another cyst that had grown straight back after my first surgery, so Mr P decided to remove it before we went ahead with any fertility treatment. Another laparoscopy was duly booked in, but as I came round from the anaesthetic, I woozily looked up to see Mr P already at my side with news: it turned out this was a nasty little cyst and was actually on the opposite side to the one they'd thought. It was so heavy it had twisted one of my Fallopian tubes and severely hampered the other. No wonder we'd not managed to get pregnant. But within three weeks of that op, you burst into life in Mummy's tummy as a little bunch of fast-dividing cells ... life's little Lego building blocks of my perfect, perfect boy.

I've already said I'm a bit of a control freak and my approach to getting pregnant involved a lot of sticks that you had to wee on! You will never get to understand this as a boy, but there is something quite compulsive about it. You can get one lot that tell you when it's the right time to try for a baby and another that reveals whether you've made one or not. In those long months waiting for you to appear I peed on hundreds of the things. I always picked the pregnancy tests where two pink lines had to appear to indicate a win in the game of baby bingo, and I always wanted more time to assess the result, squinting at it in all forms of light. There was some kind of exquisite torture in the 'Could it be a faint line? Maybe? No …' uncertainty that was oddly addictive and far preferable to those digital-style tests with their rude and very final shouts of 'NOT PREGNANT'.

But on that one magical day in early January of 2015, I picked up the test from the side of the bath after the required three-minute wait to a jolt of shock. There was no mistaking those two perfect pink lines, no squinting and tilting at the light, and I burst into absolute floods of happy, joyful, relieved, thankful tears. I rushed back into the bedroom where Daddy was still in bed, he clocked the tears and began the process of comforting me and giving it the 'next month' speech. But before he could get into full flow I shoved the pee stick with its two lines right under his nose!! He was elated and there followed the obligatory, male of the species, cheering lap around the room as he celebrated first his virility and second our happy news! That moment is up there with the best of my life. We could not have been happier that you were on your way to meet us. Should you wish to check it out for yourself I've even kept the test in your little box of baby things! Gross? Don't worry, I've Googled and discovered that pee is sterile (that was after the time you peed in your own face as a newborn, but we'll get to that in the next chapter).

* * *

This time around I'd had time to prepare and had been dealing with my anxiety to make sure I was as Zen-like as possible and gave you a smooth and stress-free ride in Mummy's tummy. I'd been to cognitive-behavioural therapy to retrain my overanxious mind, I did daily mindfulness meditation and kept my life as stress-free as possible. It's a wonder you didn't pop out in full Shaolin-monk garb. You gave me no trouble in the first twelve weeks – the first 'trimester'. I've always had a stomach of iron, I can read in cars and not get sick, and I could count on one hand the number of times I've been sick in my adult life. So, there were none of the dreaded dashes to the toilet like many pregnant women suffer. Smells didn't make me nauseous, I didn't go off coffee or tea, although I'd already cut out caffeine as part of the 'Zen experiment'. I was a bit tired, though really I mostly just used that as an excuse to get Daddy to wait on me hand and foot, a super habit that 'we' decided to stick with after you were born. I also mostly craved beige foods like crisps, chips and potatoes, but I kind of do that at the best of times anyway, and every time I tried to persuade your dad I had a 'craving' for crisps or the like, he batted me down with a 'that's a hankering not a craving'! I did do my best to get plenty of good nutrients into my system as well, as I was growing a strapping little boy (not that I knew yet whether you were a boy or a girl). Drinking during pregnancy was still a debatable issue at the time, particularly in the early stages, so I avoided alcohol through the whole nine months apart from one glass of bubbles at Auntie Jo and Uncle James's wedding and one at my baby shower in Manchester.

The dreaded twelve-week scan moment rolled around again. We were at a different hospital, Stepping Hill in Stockport, this time as I was under 'consultant-led care' because of our previous problems and loss. I had chosen to go with the aforementioned Mr P, as we had built up a relationship and he had such a wonderful, kind, calm and reassuring manner. He always put me and my concerns at ease. We'd already had a couple of early scans at seven and nine weeks to check in on you and you'd had a good, strong heartbeat both times. So, the scene for the scan was different and I felt different. Positive and oh so happy. This time it was smiles all round, the fuzzy-grey scan picture was chosen (you'll find it in your baby book) and we skipped out of there hugging and kissing and totally, totally thrilled.

We could finally share the news with the wider world – Team Bland was expanding! As you'll have gathered with this book, I am a sharer and so, after all that we'd been through, your fuzzy scan picture went straight up on Facebook. Friends and family – particularly those who knew what we'd been through the year before – couldn't have been more pleased. There was already a lot of love around for you.

Then there was the long wait in that in-between stage before we could see you again on the twenty-week scan and I would check out your growing progress in my tummy a million times a day! You had definitely formed a small bump by twelve weeks, but only that I could notice – anyone else would have thought it was just a big lunch. I stocked up on all the baby books and apps for my phone, so I could read how you were developing each week. I would read and reread each week's info with excitement. Most of them have a strange habit of comparing the baby to the size of fruit. I believe at this stage you were kind of kiwi-sized!

I so wanted a bump to show off and was one of those women who was desperate to get into maternity clothes. As I've said, any excuse for a bit of shopping. And by around sixteen weeks I was in maternity jeans and fitted tops sticking you out in my tummy for all I was worth. I often found that hands rested on the tummy were the finishing touch, as if to say to anyone looking on, yes, yes it's a baby in there, not just fat! This desperate wish for a massive pregnancy belly would come back to bite me in the end though, as after about thirty weeks I was MASSIVE! I always say you go one of two ways when pregnant – Kim or Kate. If you're small like Kim Kardashian and me, then baby will show everywhere, you retain water and end up with cankles and a fat face. Or if you're long, lean and athletic like Kate Middleton, you can stand face on to people at nine months and they won't even notice you're pregnant. I was like a ship in full sail, Freddie, but I wore it with pride for you. I even retained water in my lips! My face looks so odd in our first pictures together.

As you were due in September, I was also heavily pregnant during the long, hot summer through which I spent much of my time sweating. At work I jealously guarded the personal Dyson fan I'd been provided with, while at our roastingly hot NCT 'training for childbirth' classes, where I was more polite as we'd only just met our new friends, I only cried inwardly if someone moved a fan in a different direction. I even bought a paddling pool in which to stand my hot fat feet in the garden. Am I painting a beautiful picture of pregnant Mummy here?! But I loved every moment of carrying you around in my tummy.

In the early stages of pregnancy there is a bit of a disconnect, as you know there's a baby in there, but you can't quite see or feel it. It can feel quite unreal. But as you get nearer to halfway, you can start to feel movement. And I first felt you move in my tummy at seventeen weeks. I remember it like it was yesterday. I had just gone into Studio 11 at BBC 5 Live ready to read the news on the mid-morning show and was sat down, headphones on and poised for the top-of-the-hour jingle. Then you totally caught me by surprise as I felt you move – it was so gentle that if I'd been walking about I might have missed it. But I didn't – it felt like someone had gently rolled a marble across the inside of my tummy. I put my hand there to touch you back. Hello, little baby. I don't remember what the top story was, but I know I read it with a huge smile on my face.

A few weeks later came our twenty-week scan. It's the one where everyone asks, 'Will you find out the sex?', but is in fact more about checking for any foetal anomalies. Obviously, our main concern was checking you were shipshape in my tummy, but we had also already decided that we wanted to find out if you were a boy or a girl. A lot of people wait until the baby arrives but I'm not a huge fan of surprises. I like to be able to plan ahead and imagine how things will look in the future. They say mother's intuition is often the best predictor in the myriad unscientific ways of guessing the sex of the baby and I really thought you were a boy. And I wanted a boy. Grandad Hodges had died the previous July and it just seemed fitting that as one boy went out of the family then the next should come in.

The radiographer couldn't really have hidden it anyway as you were in my tummy in a sitting position for the scan, head by my ribs and bottom at the bottom (a place you would frustratingly decide to stay), and there was no missing you were a boy! Both Daddy and I were overjoyed. He would have been happy either way as well, but I know that because he'd always had such a wonderful relationship with Grumpy, he so wanted a son that he could recreate that love with. You are very lucky to have him as your daddy and it gives me so much comfort to know you will grow up bathed in that love and affection from him.

The rest of the pregnancy was pretty plain sailing (ship in full sail, remember?) with one tiny exception. You remained resolutely in that sitting position with your head up under my ribs. This is what is medically termed 'breech' position, and it meant if you'd decided to start heading out, it would have been feet first, making for a much more dangerous delivery. Head down is the way every baby needs to be to make being born as easy as possible. In first pregnancies it's quite common for the baby to sit like you were, then at some point perform an acrobatic forward roll to point in the right direction. You grew bigger and bigger and your movements became so obvious I could see your little fists kneading the inside of my tummy and pushing funny little lumps out in the skin of my bump. Even Daddy was able to sit with his hands on my tummy feeling you move around. Bodie also took to sitting next to me on the sofa every night and resting his nose on you under the bump – your best doggy pal right from the very start.

But through all this time I always felt your little head bobbing around under my ribs and your feet kicking away at my pelvic floor. At every midwife's check-up they kept telling me there was plenty of time for you to move. But you stuck fast – already flexing your now obvious will of iron (another trait from Mummy). I'd been through all those boiling-hot NCT birthing classes, though we were mainly there to make friends with others having babies at the same time! And ever the conscientious mother-to-be I'd signed up to a second set of earth-mother-style classes with my friend Sarah, where we'd all sit cross-legged and talk about 'breathing the baby out'. But I couldn't fully focus because I knew you just weren't budging from your breech position.

Desperate measures were needed. A spot of Googling came up with a few natural things to try. So, the final few weeks of pregnancy were spent with me kneeling on the edge of the sofa and trying to manoeuvre us into upside-down positions for ten minutes at a time. Didn't work. I tried bouncing on a large blow-up ball. Nada. Then things got really desperate and we tried the ancient Chinese trick of moxibustion. I was having acupuncture to relax at the time, so it didn't seem that outlandish a thing to try and I got all the tips from my acupuncturist. It basically involves burning a cigar-like stick of Chinese herbs called moxa next to an acupuncture point on the outside of the little toe. Obviously, at this point I couldn't reach my own knees owing to the huge bump you were making, let alone my toes, so the job of holding this boiling-hot stick of herbs as close to my toe as possible without burning the skin fell to Daddy. The odd cross word was exclaimed from my prone position on the sofa if he lost concentration … 'TOO HOT!!' We did this for ten minutes a day, every evening for two weeks and the only result was that our house smelt like some sort of drug den. You stayed firmly in place, still not keen to view the world from upside down.

The only other option left was a medical intervention known as an ECV – external cephalic version. It involves going into hospital and the doctors literally grabbing the baby through the tummy and pushing it into the head-down position. Plenty of people have it safely but to me it just sounded too invasive. There is a small risk of complications and the success rate with first babies was relatively low. I just felt you were happy in your head-up spot for a reason and if you were happy there, then I was happy with you there. I had also by this point long given up on the 'breathing the baby out' birthing malarkey and hypno-birthing CDs, and was wholly unprepared for a natural labour anyway. So we packed them away with the expensive TENS machine (apparently meant to help during labour by delivering little electric pulses known as 'transcutaneous electrical nerve stimulation' that aid contractions) which couldn't go back to the shop as Daddy had decided to open it and test it out on his arm …

It was decided: you would make your arrival on an operating table through the 'sunroof'!

Chapter 7

FRED MAKES HIS ENTRANCE

All was in place for my C-section, but obviously for us Blands there was one final drama! After choosing Mr P as the trusted man to deliver you, we went for an appointment with him a couple of weeks before the op date only to be told by one of the nurses that he was moving to a different hospital. There were a few panicked texts from me to him – I'm sure he rued the day he ever gave me his phone number! – and it was settled that he could deliver you on his first day in the new job at Wythenshawe Hospital.

We hastily arranged a tour of the facilities at the place where you were now to be born and were pleasantly surprised by what we saw. The date was arranged for 16 September – we actually got to decide your birthday! We turned up that morning not 100 per cent sure what we'd find as it was Mr P's first day in theatre. We were shown into a large room to wait to be called.

We of course arrived laden with bags and junk, knowing that I'd be staying in after the C-section. I took advantage of not having to go through a sweaty labour and had curled my hair and put make-up on – there had to be some upsides to all the breech hassle! So, we sat in our room eating sweets and reading magazines. At one point I got a little nervous when one of the nurses seemed to know nothing of Mr P, and got a bit worried that some complete stranger would be delivering my precious boy, as I did not want that! You needed to be in safe hands. But then in he strode, reassuring as ever, and said he was having a bit of a tussle with another consultant over who got to use the operating theatre first, but we'd soon be under way. A good bit of first-day consultant wars to make things interesting.

Nerves slightly calmed, I then spent the rest of the morning going to the loo every two minutes until a nurse appeared with a gown for me and blue scrubs for your dad and we were off to prep for theatre. It was a slightly odd scenario as I sat on the bed chatting to the theatre staff and waiting for the epidural to take effect. The nurse who was writing all the details of the procedure up on the whiteboard had to ask me how to spell Mr P's name! I felt in quite a position of responsibility. Then he appeared, scrubbed up and ready to go, introduced himself to all the other members of the team and we were set. First job in the new post, let's bring baby Freddie into the world, Mr P!

As you can imagine, having a baby plucked from your tummy is a slightly odd feeling. I lay flat with Daddy at my head stroking my hair and holding my hand. They put up a large blue medical sheet at the top of your tummy, so you don't have to see what's happening at the business end. However, the large theatre light fitting above my head had an unfortunate mirror effect and every so often I'd catch a glimpse and have to quickly avert my eyes! I couldn't feel a thing when the incision was made. As Mr P chatted away, all relaxed, I started to experience a very annoying side effect of the epidural, which can happen to some people, in that I began to shake uncontrollably like I'd been hiking through the Arctic. It made holding any sensible conversation very difficult as my teeth were chattering at quite some volume. So, I gave up on the talking and let Daddy take over who remarkably, with his past history of fainting in any kind of gory medical situation, was totally relaxed and happy.

I was told to expect some sensation of movement 'a bit like a washing machine', then suddenly from behind the blue sheet came a high-pitched cry. You had arrived! And you were making your presence known to the world in full-lunged fashion. It was and is the most wonderful moment of my life and was such a strange mix of emotions. I was immediately totally choked up with tears streaming down my quivering, chattering face. It sounds a weird thing to say, having carried you around in my tummy for nine months, feeling you move, playing you music and stroking your head as it bulged out of my bump, but it was only at that moment I felt, 'Oh wow, it's actually a baby, it's real'. I was obviously stuck on the operating table as they whisked you over to the scales to rub you down and weigh you, but it was immediately clear to me why you had defiantly stayed in that breech position. The first thing I noticed was your enormously long legs! They were huge – well, long and skinny like your dad's. No wonder you couldn't somersault in my tummy with those in the way. I quickly congratulated myself on not putting you through that ECV.

The second thing I noticed and exclaimed at was your hair! Grandma had always gone on about babies on our side of the family being fair, but you had loads of thick dark-brown hair and it looked beautiful. I gazed over at you on the other side of the theatre already totally in love with the little boy who Daddy and I had created together. It was 12.36 p.m. on Wednesday 16 September 2015 and you, our little legend, weighed in at 7 lb 4 oz or 3,305 grams and measured a top length of 56 cm – most of it leg.

Having known you were a boy since the twenty-week scan we had already decided on your name. We'd each put together our own shortlist of three names each and both included Freddie. It was a name each of us loved; our families did too and there are ancestors called Frederick on both Mummy's and Daddy's side of the family. Whether you are officially Freddie or Frederick is a little conundrum I shall come to later. Another case of Mummy not being able to make up her mind! Your first middle name, David, was in honour of Grandad Hodges of course and your second, Jackson, is a surname from Grumpy's family, which they now often use as a middle name, so a nod to both sides of your heritage.

Once all the particulars were noted and you were wrapped up in a hospital-issue blue baby blanket and little yellow woollen hat, you were brought back over to us. Daddy was actually the first to hold you as I was still shaking fairly uncontrollably and was worried about dropping you! He had such a look of pride on his face as he gazed down at you, our beautiful new son. You had blue/grey eyes, one of which was stuck slightly shut for the first few hours, that mop of dark-brown hair and your long legs. As is common after a baby has been sitting breech your legs popped up next to your sides frog-like in a little M-shape. They would stay like that for quite a few weeks refusing to be pushed into the legs of a Babygro! Your face, having not had to go through the traumatic squeezing process of natural labour, was totally perfectly formed. You looked much as you do now. In fact I've just shown you the first picture of you now and asked, 'Who's that?' Your reply? 'Baby Freddie'!

If you consult your baby book that I studiously filled in over your first year, you'll find the weather on the day you were born was dry and sunny, a good omen I hope for a sunshine-filled life ahead. Teenage heart-throb Justin Bieber was at No. 1 in the charts with 'What Do You Mean?', David Cameron was the Tory Prime Minister and Queen Elizabeth II was on the throne. That's something I'm pretty sure will have changed by the time you're reading this yourself. As ever in this life, time moves on, history is left behind and the future rolls relentlessly forward.

* * *

I was stitched up and sent into recovery where I finally got to hold you for the first time. It was quite a struggle to get you out of Daddy's arms! But as soon as you nestled into my chest, my tiny little snuggly Fred, it was like you were always meant to be there. And I knew I loved you more than anything in the world. It was both a soft and gentle kind of love and a fierce one too. I would do anything for my precious boy.

Time in recovery seemed a bit of a blur. Midwives popped in and out, I made an attempt at breastfeeding you which seemed to go okay and we had lots of skin-on-skin cuddles. At one point, an hour or so in, just as we thought we were old pros, we got told off by a nurse for not having enough layers on you. Because we were coping so well we got left there for a bit and your first visitors were allowed to see us there. In trooped Grandma, Gran and Grumpy, all totally delighted with their gorgeous new grandson. We recorded the happy moment with photos for posterity and then I got Daddy onto the really important job of the day … getting me a private room!

I've never been one for sharing rooms. I am such a light sleeper that the smallest sound will wake me and then I'll worry about tossing and turning and keeping other people awake. Sharing beds with friends on teenage sleepovers was my idea of hell and so it made sense that if I had to stay overnight at hospital, especially with my new little Fred to look out for, then it needed to be in a private room. I'm also not big on shared bathroom facilities and I didn't want to be walking miles down a corridor to the loo while holding onto my new C-section stitches, so the draw of an en-suite bathroom was pretty high up there too. I'd been through a pretty major surgery, so I thought I'd earned this small luxury. I was the last of our NCT group to give birth and I'd heard some wild and wonderful tales of goings-on on the maternity ward. The private rooms you could pay for if they were free and I was DETERMINED to get one. It was like I was going for the trophy at Wimbledon! But there was a tournament to be played first … you couldn't book ahead and must already be on the way up to the ward before the private room of one's dreams could be allocated.

So, as I sat cuddling you in the recovery bed, I had to enlist Daddy as a doubles' partner and all my conversation with him centred on him asking the nurse about a private room, then asking the nurse when I was on the way up to the ward, so we could ask again there. Then telling him to just get up to the ward and get me the room! It was a full-on hormone fuelled-FOMO moment. I get a lot of Fear Of Missing Out, something I hope you won't have inherited. It's a high-stakes, high-stress pastime that invariably ends in disappointment! Just as poor Daddy was beginning to lose that new-father happy glow and look a bit frazzled by my constant room requests, a private room was found and secured, and we could all relax up in our new digs on the maternity ward.

Having now spent many a night in hospital, I can say a private room is just as good as any hotel. You have a super-snug bed with an electric control to whizz it into the most comfortable position, clean sheets and blankets and a huge en-suite with a chair in the shower. What more could a new mum want?! And nobody to keep me awake. Or so I thought …

We spent a lovely first evening together in that room. We cleaned up your thatch of dark hair with a sponge, popped on your tiny newborn nappy and got out your first little Babygro to wear that we had lovingly chosen and packed up especially. There must be something special they put in the cotton of a Babygro, or maybe it's just the feeling when they're on a warm little newborn, but they are the softest garments known to man. This little one had grey-and-white stripes and little elephants on it, and despite being newborn-sized and you being a relatively long baby it totally swamped you. And those little breech froggy legs kept slipping out of the trousers. As you lay on your back in the little plastic cot they had put in the room, we snapped your first photo that we would send out to the world, or the world of social media at least. You are holding your hands up as if conducting an orchestra – and I know every parent thinks this, but you were hands down the cutest little baby in town.

Daddy was given the important job of revealing your arrival to the world on Facebook. Some new parents wait a few days for this big announcement, some never even make it on a public forum. But we are sharers and were so enthralled by you that we waited less than four hours after your birth to share you with a wider public. So, at 6.16 p.m. the crazy 'baby musical conductor' photo was posted with the following proud message:

> Everyone, meet Freddie! Freddie David Jackson Bland was born at 12.36 this afternoon weighing 7 lb 4 oz. He's a little belter with a cracking head of hair. Mum and baby are doing great. So proud of Rachael Bland!!

And of course, just like us, the people adored you.

* * *

The evening passed by in a blur. I was still semi-paralysed from the epidural and had been cut through every layer of my tummy, which made shifting around in bed a little tricky. But Daddy was on hand to alternately pass me you, drinks, sandwiches and my phone. I'd heard from some of the other NCT girls who'd had C-sections that they'd been told not to try and get out of bed to pick up the baby and that a midwife would be on hand to pass baby over when it needed feeding or attention. I'd also been told that newborns sleep very heavily the first couple of nights as they're very tired from their arduous journey through birth. Both of these 'facts' turned out to be absolute nonsense.

But it was labouring under these misapprehensions that I finally allowed Daddy to go home to enjoy his celebratory whiskey and toast his newborn son at around 11 p.m. I called the nurse for some painkillers and settled back in the bed thinking I'd catch up on some sleep after my busy first day as a new mum! And there came my first lesson as a parent: you will never have time to relax by yourself again.

Almost the second your daddy had stepped out of the door, you started crying, and there didn't appear to be a way of stopping you. Now rather inconveniently the private room was quite big, with the bed in the middle and your cot pushed up against a wall that was a good two metres away. Not that far, you may think, but it was like running a marathon to get up and out of bed, then move across the room to pick up 7 lb of squirmy little boy while holding on to the C-section stitches!

No midwives magically appeared to help out so there was nothing for it but to keep making that trip back and forth to try and settle you. This was interspersed with cuddling you in the bed and attempting more breastfeeding. At one point I actually thought I had the whole thing nailed. But then the hours just kept on ticking by and there was no sign of you going to sleep. Turns out coming out through the sunroof isn't as tiring as a standard delivery.

* * *

From the very earliest stage in your life it became apparent that hats would never be your thing. You are blessed with what I'll call a 'fine' head from your mummy. Remember that yellow hat they put on you as soon as you were born? We carelessly cast that aside in the recovery area, swapping it for one of our expensive shop-bought ones, a decision we came to regret. The little woollen ones at the hospital are perfectly sized to stay put on a teeny newborn head. A shop-bought cotton number, while perhaps looking smarter, is very much not. While trying to feed you, I spent most of the time pushing that damn hat up out of your eyes and wishing we'd held on to the yellow knitted number. This set the tone for you and hats, and as soon as you had the ability to use your hands to whip them off your head then you would! Even now you refuse to wear a hat in the sun. Unless it's a fireman's hat of course, and then you won't take it off!

Your wailing went up a notch and in turns I naturally started trying the things that I would later read in baby books are standard ways to settle a fussy baby. I tried shush shush shushing you from my bed. That would work a little. Then a genius idea – there was a washbasin in the corner of the room with the tap on a timer. So, a large part of the night was spent slumped up against the wall in the corner wildly waving a hand across the sensor, as the gushing of the water seemed to have a calming effect on your crying. In later weeks I discovered you could simply download an app with all these baby-soothing sounds on and you'd happily drift off to the noise of a 'babbling brook'!

There were moments where I felt totally on top of motherhood that night. I'd been so worried in the lead-up to your birth that I wouldn't be a good mother or know what to do. And most of the time I didn't have a clue, but I knew how much I loved you and that was all that mattered. I fired off a few texts to Daddy in the wee small hours. Visiting started at 9 a.m. and in my quest to avoid all hospital food, I asked him if he could stop off at Costa Coffee on the way in and grab us breakfast. But then as the night carried on with you not sleeping, me hauling my now rather stiff body in and out of the hospital bed back and forth to your cot, while waving a hand under the tap sensor, my texts to Daddy took on a more desperate tone.

First (I think this was around 4 a.m.) came the call to drop the Costa trip and just get here for 9. Then an hour later, something along the lines of 'I DON'T CARE WHAT TIME VISITING STARTS JUST GET HERE AS SOON AS YOU WAKE UP!!!!' Of course, all these texts went unanswered until he replied at around 8 a.m. saying, 'Gosh sorry, only just got all these, I was asleep as soon as my head hit the pillow'. Probably not the best response under my sleep-deprived circumstances.

At some point around 5 a.m. one of the midwives had finally appeared and immediately took pity on my wild-eyed banshee-looking face. She patiently explained that a lot of new babies don't like the feeling of sleeping on their backs in a cot, as it is so different from being snuggled up all warm in the womb, and so she rolled up some baby blankets, tucked them around you and as if by magic you went to sleep. Finally, a little rest for a tired mummy, though only for an hour or so until we were rudely awakened by an early call from a nurse who'd come for her routine check on your hearing. At 7 a.m. They have no mercy in hospital.

* * *

Luckily, by the time Daddy had arrived just after 9, with the aforementioned Costa, my night-time troubles seemed a million miles away and we were happily ensconced in our parental bliss again. However, the night's trials hadn't fully left me, and I was determined to return home. Back when Grandma had a C-section with Uncle Matthew they kept her in hospital for ten days! Not any more. I'd heard there was a 'fast-track' path out where you could get home in twenty-four hours and with Mummy's competitive spirit if I wasn't home in time for dinner that night, then I would not have been happy.

I passed all the necessary tests – walking, weeing, getting dressed – and I was primed and ready to go. I'd been pretty chuffed with my attempts at breastfeeding overnight and felt really quite proficient. It was something I absolutely wanted to do to give you the best nutritional start in life, but the idea pre-birth had kind of freaked me out. So, feeling like I was nailing it came as a pleasant surprise. That is until the breastfeeding police arrived and tried to undermine me. The nurses told me they weren't sure you were getting enough and latching on properly, and while one manhandled a boob another said they thought I should stay in another night, so they could supervise.

I refused. I was on the fast-track, remember? I knew I had this breastfeeding under control and could do a much better job left to my own devices at home. I knew if I stayed, my confidence would be dented and a lot of motherhood is about trusting your own intuition. So, not for the last time, I declined another night at the Hotel Hospital and signed myself out.

We didn't manage to escape before being ambushed by the 'newborn photography' lady. With hindsight this kind of thing shouldn't be allowed when you're high on hormones and newborn love. She basically arrives pushing a cart sponsored by some baby product or other, offering to take some very average pictures of you and your newborn for a not insubstantial amount of money! We'd turned her away once, but she was wily and persisted and by the time she arrived back we were all cock-a-hoop about going home and allowed her into the family circle. You look beautiful in the pictures, of course, but the ones of me are not my best. I'm wearing a nursing bra and nursing vest and have not been caught at a flattering angle. Because we spent so much on those pictures it then seemed a bit wasteful to go for another newborn shoot at a proper photography studio. I always kind of hankered after one of those stylized pictures of you snuggled up in a woollen bear-ears bonnet in a knitted basket. With that image in mind, I imagine you are thanking your lucky stars the average hospital photographer got to us first!

Chapter 8

PARENTING – A CRASH COURSE IN BABY POO

Taking your newborn baby home from hospital is a bit like driving a car on your own for the first time after you pass your test. You feel nervous, exhilarated and not wholly in control. There is the checking-out process from the ward where they make sure you're going home in the regulation car seat and then, bam, you are unleashed on the world with your new charge fully under your care.

I had planned your 'going-home outfit' with precision. This is something I've always done with your clothes, as I love for you to be well turned out and you can rock a great toddler style these days. With hindsight, for the journey home I may have over-accessorized you. There was the White Company koala Babygro, with matching grey-and-white striped hat. I loved a grey-and-white stripe! Then a cute little blue-and-white striped, chunky-knit hooded cardigan. All topped off with an utterly pointless but nonetheless cute pair of furry White Company koala booties. Yep, you were pretty much swamped by fabric – and underneath the newborn insert in the car seat and added blanket it's a wonder you didn't overheat on the way home.

For Freddie

How many layers to dress a baby in will remain one of life's great mysteries to me. After that early telling-off in recovery for not having enough clothes or a hat on you I was forever perplexed. It was September and warm – did you need a hat? What about a blanket, or two? A vest under a Babygro? Did you need scratch mittens? The answer to this one is always no, by the way. They are little mittens designed to go on a tiny baby's hands, because while you had little soft fingers your nails were mighty sharp! But they are the biggest con in the world of baby clothes. There is just NO WAY the damn things will stay on wriggly little fingers. And then some sensible midwife told me that babies want to touch their faces with their hands in a self-comforting way, so they all went in the bin. When you have children, as I hope you will one day, then you will truly understand this great life conundrum.

The correct temperature has always been a bone of contention between your dad and I. He comes from two families of Cumbrian hill farmers who grew up in freezing-cold farmhouses where sticking on an extra layer was the way to get warm. Even after Gran and Grumpy moved to a centrally heated house in Knutsford they weren't big energy users, and Daddy and Auntie Claire often tell stories of being told to move around more if they complained of being cold. I also think men's bodies run on a totally different thermostat setting to those of most women. Hence the thermostat wars. I can often be found in winter nonchalantly wandering by and turning it up a few degrees, until your dad starts sweating, notices and turns it down again. I've always really felt the cold. I have terrible circulation and borderline Raynaud's syndrome where the blood will often drain from my fingers in the cold leaving my nails blue. Your dad always laughs at me when I tell him I am 'cold to my very core'! So it was no surprise that as soon as you and your puzzling layers of clothes arrived, if I dressed you, there would

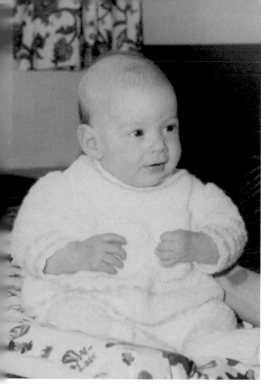

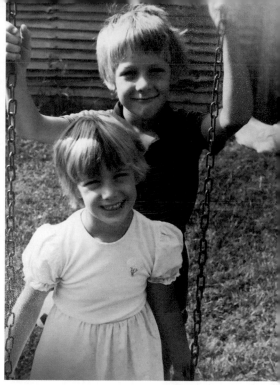

Mummy, aged four months, in the Creigiau house where Grandma and Grandad have lived ever since.

Mummy and Uncle Matthew in the garden, swinging to our hearts' content, in summer 1982.

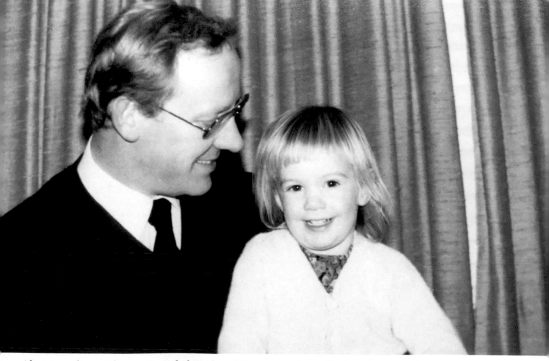

Always smiling with your Grandad Hodges. He was wearing a black tie because this photo was taken very shortly after the death of his brother, Uncle Bob, in December 1979.

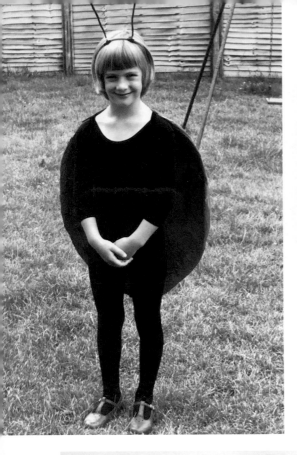

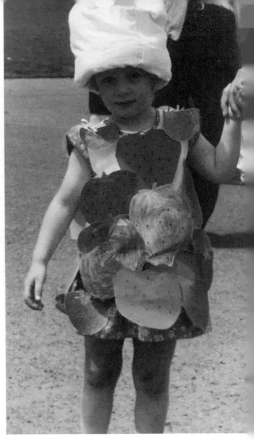

Dressed up and ready to
go to Creigiau Carnival,
as a ladybird (*left*) and
Strawberries and Cream
(*right*).

Enjoying the simple things
in life with Emma, our
friends' dog.

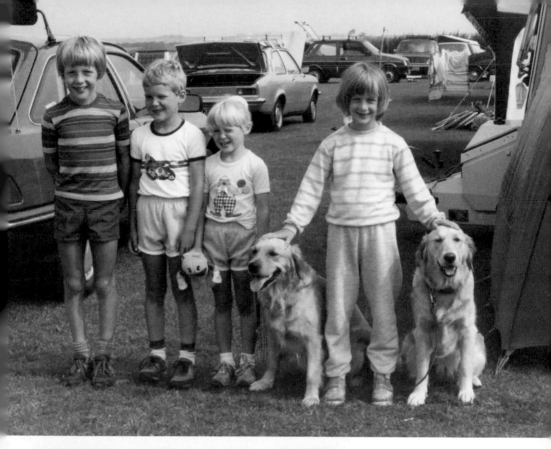

One of our many family trips to Devon with more furry companions. Our friends' dog Emma is on the left and our first dog Sophie is on the right.

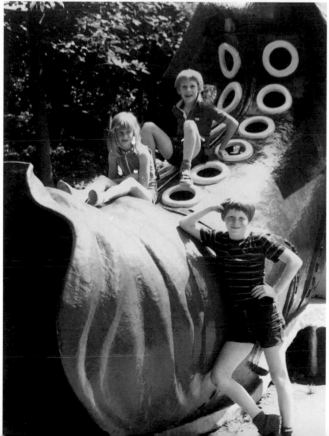

Summer silliness with Uncle Matthew and my cousin Robbie on the Isle of Wight.

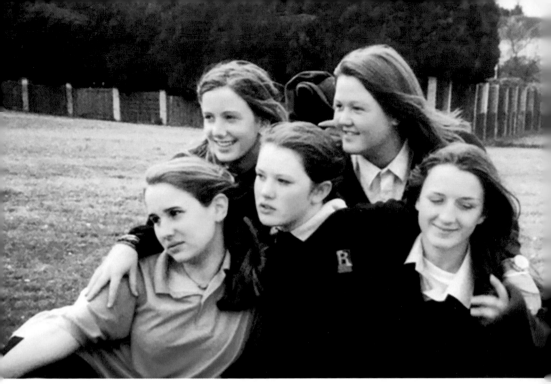

Ready for our album cover! Schooldays, 1994.

In my happy place, with Grandad watching Formula 1 at Spa in Belgium. This was our first F1 trip of many!

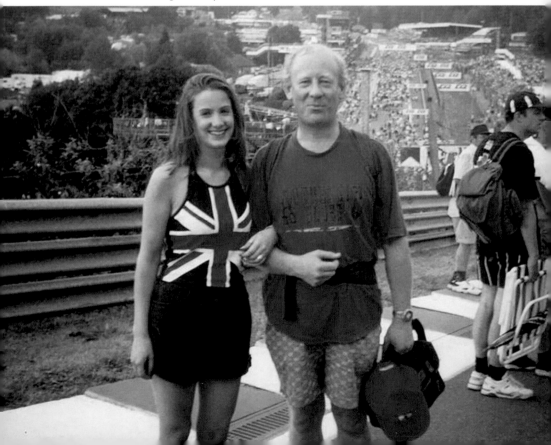

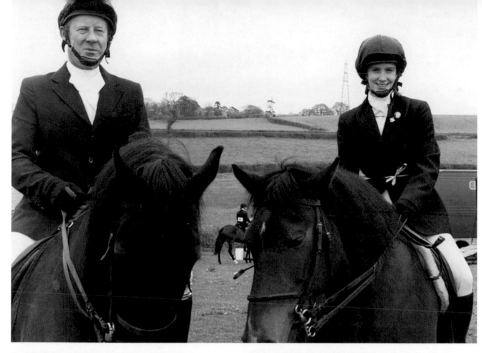

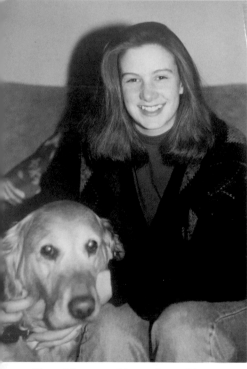

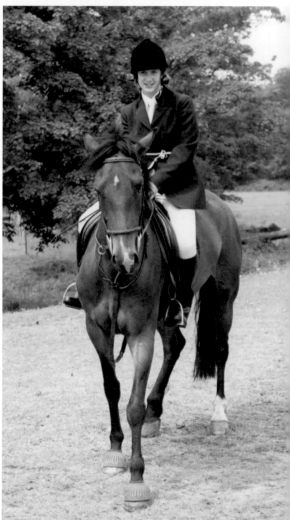

Above: Mummy with our first golden retriever, Sophie.

Top: My love for horses would last for the rest of my life. Your mummy with Grandad Hodges, all set for show day.

Right: Mummy and her beloved horse, Cariad.

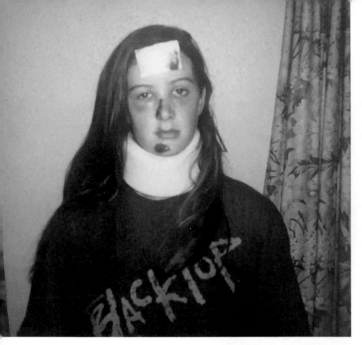

The aftermath of the car accident in 1994, which changed my life for ever.

Left to right: Mummy, Julia, Kat, Rachael. My university mates – friends for a lifetime.

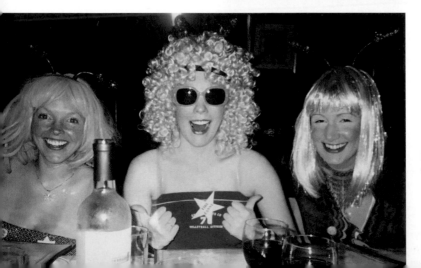

Playing dress-up with my uni girls.

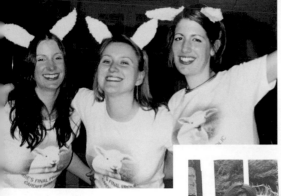

Mummy with uni girls Julia and Kat at Rachael's hen do.

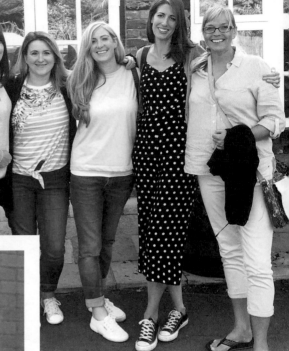

University reunion. We haven't changed a bit!

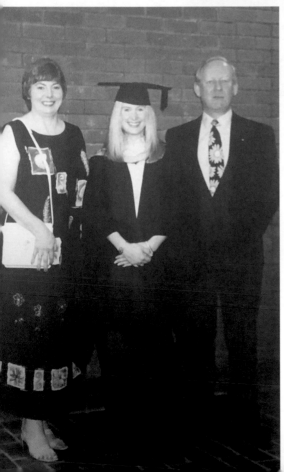

A very proud day: graduating from my postgrad course in Preston, with Grandma and Grandad Hodges by my side, in July 2001.

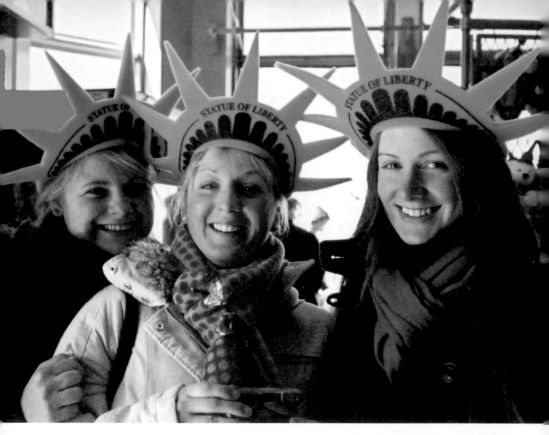

Blending in with the locals on the infamous holiday to New York in 2004.

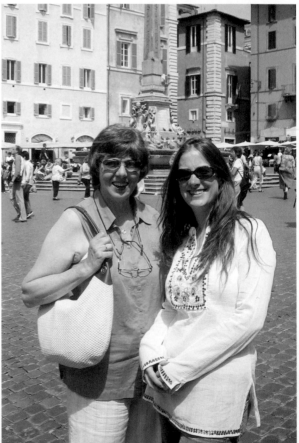

Grandma and Mummy in Rome for Grandma's sixtieth birthday in 2005. Grandma had never flown before this trip!

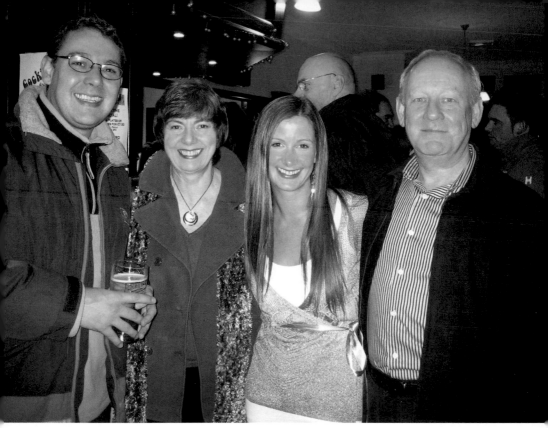

The family all together, Christmas Eve 2007.

Mummy's first permanent job at the BBC. This was me with my BBC Swindon and Wiltshire *Drive* co-presenter, Mark Jones.

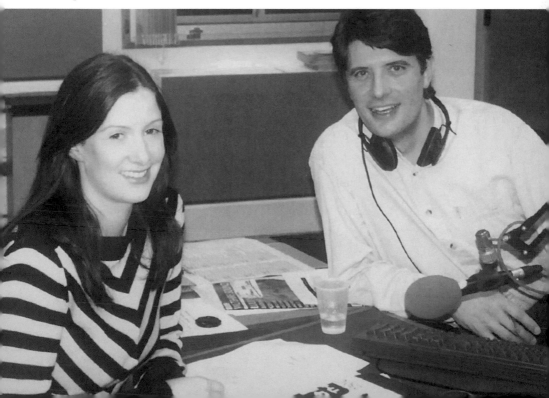

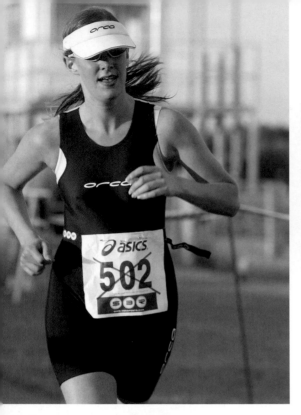

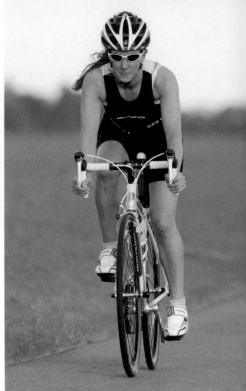

I never thought I'd be an athlete, let alone one who could do a triathlon! This took place at Eton Dorney Lake.

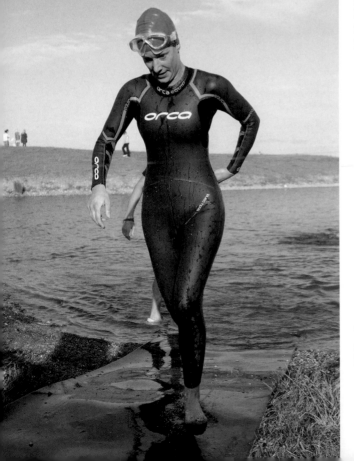

The finish line: a very proud moment, which reignited my love of exercise.

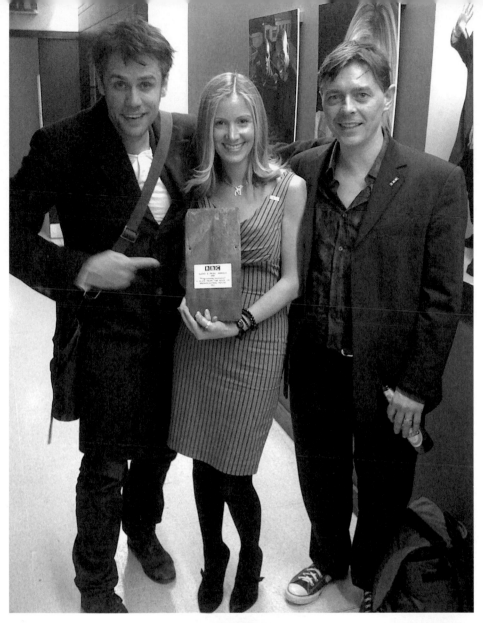

Winning the Programming Innovation category at the Audio and Music Awards. The award was a slate from the roof of the original Broadcasting House.

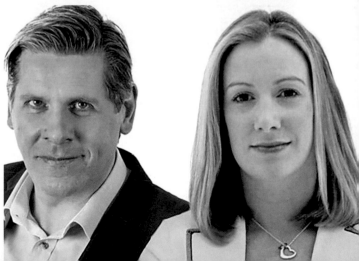

Publicity shot for 5 Live with the incomparable and fabulous Tony Livesey.

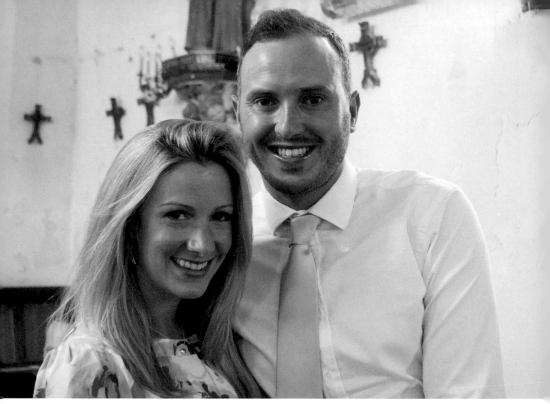

Mummy and Daddy together at a wedding in France. Don't we scrub up well?!

A very special night, when Daddy asked me to marry him – onesies and all.

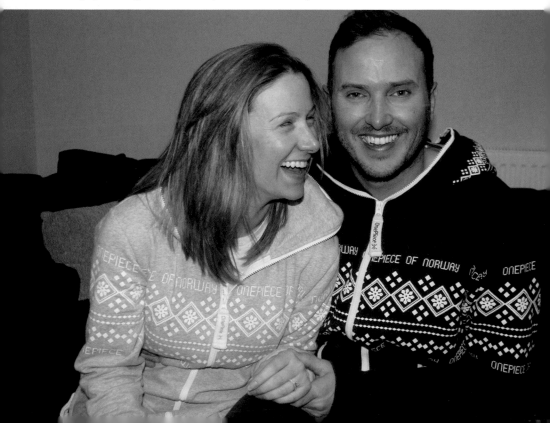

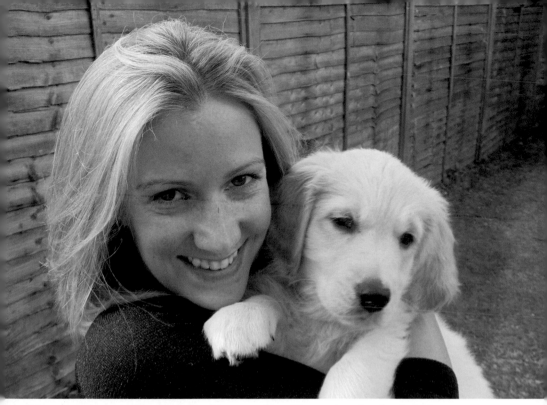

Mummy with your pal Bodie, during his puppy days. He was a heartbreaker from day one.

My all-time musical hero Brandon Flowers, from The Killers, actually wrote me a birthday card!

Mummy tracked Brandon down when he popped into the BBC.

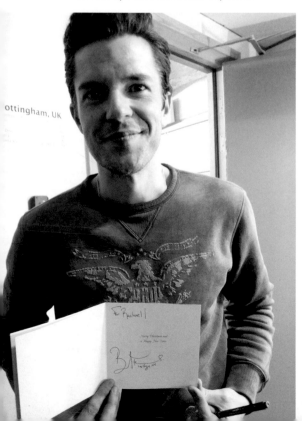

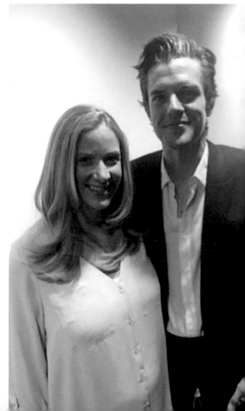

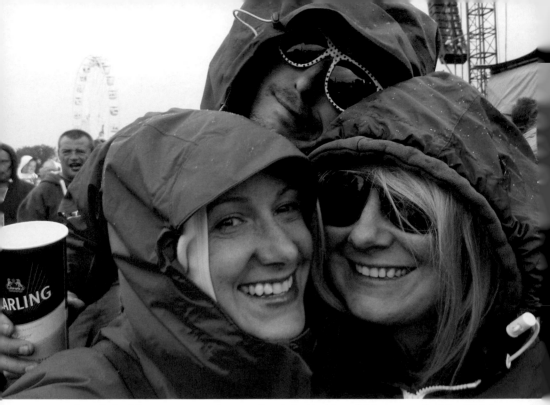

Best friends for life, come rain or shine … Auntie Jo, Daddy and Mummy at the Isle of Wight Festival in 2012.

Dancing like a loon watching The Killers in Hyde Park, 2017.

Festival beer selfie with your Auntie Jo.

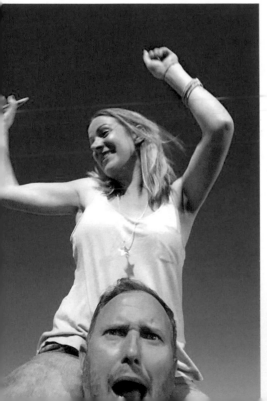

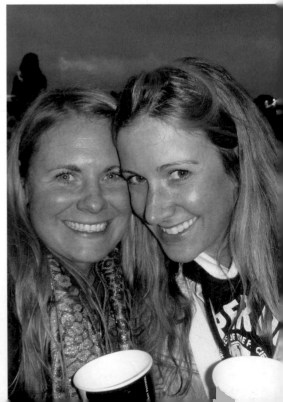

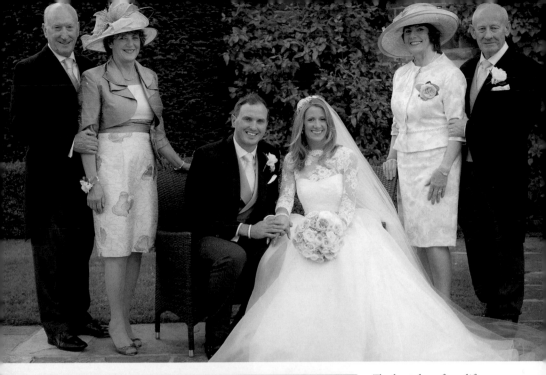

The best day of my life, apart from the day when you were born. Mummy and Daddy on our wedding day, with your proud grandparents.

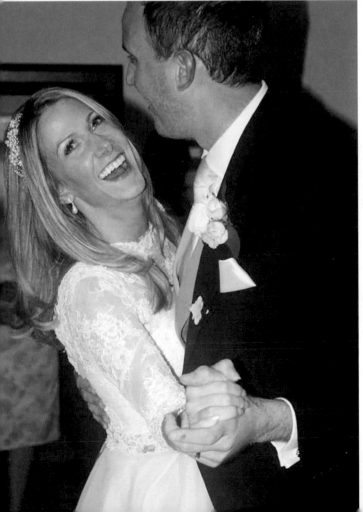

Our first dance, so full of love.

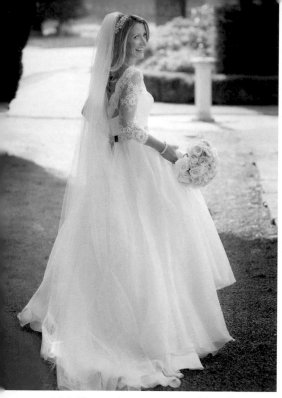

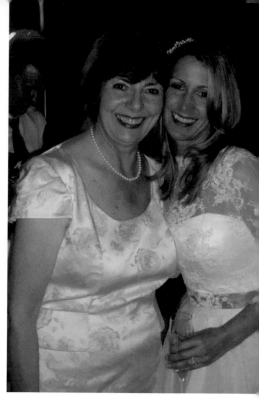

I felt like a princess on my wedding day in my beautiful dress.

Celebrating with Grandma. I couldn't have been happier.

A slightly drunken night during our honeymoon on the paradise island of Maafushivaru, in the Maldives. We were suntanned and relaxed and ready to start our life together.

I finally beat Daddy at chess!

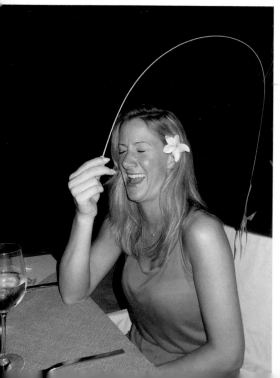

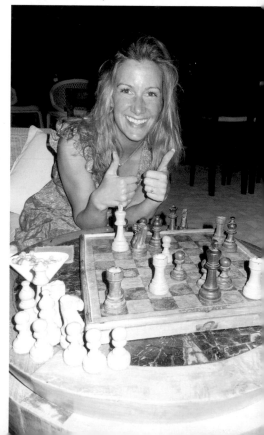

always be one extra, but if Daddy did, then there'd be one less!

We successfully navigated the journey home and crossed the threshold as our family of three. Now remember my great taste in fairly terrible films? There was another your dad and I found very funny called *The Hangover*. It's probably one to watch when you're a bit older and not the most highbrow of cultural reference points, but as soon as we got you home Daddy and I would sing a little song from it when we were having snuggles with you. It's actually sung by Zach Galifianakis's character, Alan, while travelling with his new pals in a car: 'We're the three best friends that anyone could have …'

I got Daddy a leather keyring from you for Father's Day this year that is stamped 'THREE BEST FRIENDS 16-09-15'. And even though I may not be around in person for you, my wonderful Freddie, my love will never, ever, ever leave you. Always remember that.

* * *

Those first few days at home with you passed by in a blissful bubble. It's such a topsy-turvy time where the highs of hormones and love balance out the tiredness and general sense of confusion. There was a constant stream of visitors coming and going, all so happy and thrilled to meet gorgeous baby Freddie. And you know how much Mummy loves happiness all around. I also like stuff, and wow you were a great excuse to surround ourselves with it! Suddenly your little electric rocking chair that my friends had given me at my baby shower took centre stage in the lounge, swinging you, perhaps with hindsight, a little violently back and forth! It also served the purpose of keeping you off the floor and away from a confused-looking Bodie, wondering what on earth was this little whingy bundle that had invaded his happy home. Beautiful pastel-coloured baby gifts piled up from friends and family, each one lovingly chosen and gratefully received. I felt like I knew what I was doing, I was a mummy! I'd never been the most maternal person as I'd not grown up with any younger children around. I often found I didn't know what to say to children, but as soon as I held you in my arms it felt natural and I just knew what I needed to do. I could even see Grandma was super-impressed at how good I was at this, not that she'd ever doubted me, but I could tell she was proud of the mother I had suddenly morphed into.

The nursery rhymes played, the lack of sleep made us delirious. People brought us food, there seemed to be no time frame to the days and, after a bit of Googling, I discovered if I timed it right with breastfeeding, I could even have the odd glass of bubbles. For a good week it was like being at some sort of psychedelic baby-themed festival.

Then day eight. The comedown from the hormone high hit me like a tonne of bricks. Among the constant stream of visiting friends when you have a newborn comes a constant stream of medical professionals. Now I know they have an important job to do in safeguarding babies and new mothers, but sometimes I think they can just tip you the other way. I was resolutely still breastfeeding you and determined not to top up with formula. I don't know now why I cared so much but at the time it was like a personal challenge to only grow you using the natural stuff and I can be stubborn as an ox when my mind is set on something. The problem is, you were born long and skinny and that is how you have remained. You were just never destined to be a chubby baby. You were never a big feeder as a newborn and you're still not motivated by food now. You eat when you're hungry, unless of course you spot some 'choc' on offer.

But the health system loves weighing and charts. Just moments after you were born a red book was thrust upon you, with graphs ready to be plotted into childhood. You have always been right at the bottom for weight and top for height. Long and skinny, just like your dad. But the health-system graphs don't like long and skinny. Faces were pulled, numbers were crunched and it was declared that you were close to losing ten per cent of your birthweight. It's normal for babies to lose weight in the first week while waiting for mother's milk to come out. But if you lose too much, then you are whipped back into hospital for some extra feeding. It was with this hanging over us that I had my first crisis of confidence. 'Top him up with some extra milk after feeding,' the midwife blithely said. I nodded at her vaguely, all the while in my head doing just what you do now when you don't want to do what you're told: arms crossed, face set into a frown, lips pursed with a very firm 'NO!' I of course, very politely waved her off with a smile and at 8 p.m., after eight days of little sleep, decided NOW was the time to get to grips with the dreaded piece of machinery that is the breast pump. No formula for my boy. I would make this thing work and top him up with proper milk.

Now I struggle to get your toys out of their plastic packaging, so why I had not read the instruction manual beforehand I don't know. But I took out all the parts and got to the first job of washing them in soapy water in the upstairs washbasin. But as I rinsed them off and let the water run out I realized I had washed some small but vital plastic seals down the plughole as well. Without them it wouldn't work and it felt like the end of the world! Never have so many tears been shed over a couple of small bits of plastic. But to me it was the first challenge of motherhood I deemed myself to have failed and I took it rather badly. Poor Daddy was Googling where to get replacements delivered asap, but then like any new dad in his position … he called in his own dad. And miracle of miracles Grumpy appeared with a set of the exact seals that Auntie Claire had knocking about! You, of course, were totally oblivious, and slept through the whole debacle. By the time Grumpy arrived I'd got a grip of myself and felt like a bit of a snivelling drama queen. And peace was restored to the Bland household for another night. Well, until your next feeding time of course. The moral of this story is not to put too much pressure on yourself to be perfect. Goals are good, but all of the people can't be all right all of the time. I think Bob Dylan said that.

* * *

One of the things I enjoyed most about preparing for your arrival was decorating the nursery. Your room was arbitrarily chosen as it was the last one upstairs to be decorated. It actually turned out to be the least practical room for a baby as it sits over the garage and has only a small window that opens, so it holds the heat in summer and gets freezing in winter as no heat is rising from the floor below! These were issues I had yet to discover as I threw myself into transforming the latest room in our home. If I tell you the previous owners had left it with bright-red walls and a roller blind as a door on the interior cupboard then you'll understand why neutral-loving Mummy wanted to get at it with a paintbrush and some beautiful nursery paraphernalia. Our fix-it guy Grumpy was enlisted to steam those thick layers of painted paper off the walls, a plasterer came in to skim it from top to bottom and get rid of the dreaded seventies-style Artex textured ceiling (perhaps not the worst trend from the seventies, but it's up there for me), the old stained carpet was ripped out and we were ready to create!

Now guess what colour Mummy went for …? Remember all those baby suits now … obviously a pale grey! I loved a good Farrow & Ball colour back then (a very expensive paint with beautiful depth of colour) and the grey I chose was actually called 'Cornforth White'. You'll note I don't say 'we' here. Poor Daddy didn't get much of a look-in when it came to the decorating decisions. Any attempt at input from him was generally met with an arched eyebrow and a slight shake of the head. I had 'my vision' and I was sticking to it. He did his work with Grumpy, applying the many layers of paint needed on the newly plastered walls and ceiling. In went a thick grey carpet that was beautifully soft underfoot. Grey blackout curtains with little white stars were hung from grey curtain poles and, with a bit of blood, sweat and tears, the men put together your white wooden nursery furniture. I got butterflies as I walked in and saw your cot there for the first time! You wouldn't sleep in there for a few months yet, but it was helping to make it all feel like we really were becoming parents.

I visited the RHS Flower Show at Tatton Park that year with Grandma, even though I am in no way green-fingered. I can kill a house plant from twenty paces just by looking at it, but I appreciate other people's fabulous gardens and it's a lovely day out. But barely a rose was sniffed by me or a walled water garden walked through. Nope, I spent pretty much the whole of it in the Country Living exhibition tent buying things for your nursery! I found two beautiful distressed-wood-framed pictures of cartoon owls on a pale brown background with pastel pink-and-blue accents – I thought that was a good bit of gender neutrality which was just becoming all the rage! And I bought a beautiful white embroidered quilt to put on the day bed that we would leave in your room (which would come in very handy later, on broken nights of sleep with you). White was perhaps not the best choice, and that quilt is now covered in stains of an indeterminate nature from your first year, but with a few scatter cushions on the day bed and some grey-and-white stripy boxes to hold all your newborn junk, we were nearly there. The addition of a fairly ugly but very comfortable grey-and-white nursing chair and stool created a very happy place where we would spend a lot of our time quietly feeding, rocking and snuggling. And to top off the owl theme there was a big decal sticker of an owl on a moon and a little owl-shaped night light. And so, with these last few details, your new little room was ready for you.

I adored it – it was so perfect. I would sit in there for hours before you arrived, just relaxing in my serene surroundings or rocking you in my bump on the chair, trying to imagine you in there. Then I almost got too attached. I began to think this room was really too nice to put a baby and his mess in! I've never been a big cleaner – you'll rarely find me bleaching surfaces in a pair of Marigolds – but I like a tidy home and everything in its place. But this was another of the first rules of parenthood you taught us, Freddie. You came with a lot of mess and you taught me not to be so uptight about our home looking perfect all the time. See? I was learning just as much from you about life as I was teaching you.

One of those moments when you reminded me it was always better to laugh than cry was the night of the 'poo on the curtains' incident. Now baby poo comes in all forms in the first few months and there are whole sections of mummy websites dedicated to pictures of it with questions about what's normal. And it seems when it comes to baby poo, pretty much anything goes. For a little dude you had quite some fire power and with a liquid-only diet you can imagine the potential consequences. I have never laughed so much as I did the first time I saw Daddy literally duck for cover at one of your baby farts. We'd often use a small cloth as a cover as soon as your nappy came off, as like most boys you had your own inbuilt sprinkler system. One time when I perhaps wasn't paying full attention you managed to pee in your own face, which sent me to Google whether this was a problem. But it turns out wee is sterile and actually fine to drink! Still I think it's the kind of thing best left to Bear Grylls and his camping gang.

Back to the poo though. When you would wake during the night, the deal was I was in charge of what went in and Daddy had to clean up what came out. At this point you were still tiny and slept in a SnüzPod bedside crib right next to my side of the bed. All your changing paraphernalia was stored in your still-pristine nursery where Daddy duly headed off to pop on a new nappy. Just as I was settling down to go back to sleep one night, my side of the night-time feeding ritual finished with, anguished shouts began to emanate from the nursery, followed by more panicked calling from Daddy. I dashed into the nursery to find him stood there in a state of shock with liquid baby poo all over his hands, top and the changing table. I stared at your dad for a moment, open-mouthed, then my eyes followed the poo trajectory to see it all down the side of your pristine and as yet unused white cot, and also dripping down those lovely white-and-grey starred curtains. Now if you had warned me this was going to happen when I was pregnant and shouting at anyone who dared leave a dirty fingerprint around my perfect nursery, there may have been tears. But after those few seconds of us taking in the quite frankly ridiculously grim scene, the only tears were those of proper delirious laughter. The kind of hysteria than can only be felt by two very sleep-deprived people who were now a bit 'in the shit'. It was proper doubled over, tears streaming down face, weak at the knees laughter. Well, for me anyway. Daddy couldn't hold onto anything with his hands covered in baby poo. Once I'd recovered myself to a hiccuppingly acceptable level of mirth, I began liberally chucking baby wipes and anti-bacterial spray around the place and we got stuck into the clean-up operation together. We never did quite get the stain out of those curtains, but it was one of the many moments through those early months that absolutely confirmed to me that there was no one else in the world I would rather be on that parenting rollercoaster with than your daddy. Just as long as he'd given his hands a good scrub first.

* * *

One of the big milestones for every parent in the first few weeks of having a baby is the moment it comes to register the birth of their new offspring. As I mentioned earlier we had your name all decided before you were born. Well, mostly. To me you were always a Freddie or Fred … Fredlington, Fredderico, Fredster … the pet name list goes on. The bottom line was I wanted you to be a Freddie. But Daddy and your grandparents all liked the idea of having the longer form of Frederick on your birth certificate. They argued it had more heritage and it was nice for you to have the option of the longer form. I allowed myself to be persuaded when Daddy said it would never have to be used but would just sit there on your birth certificate.

We headed into the centre of Manchester, our first big trip out with you, and into the musty old register office in Heron House. It was really like heading back into the seventies with its dated decor and piles of old books and files hanging about. We were shown into a room at the allotted appointment time for the serious legal bit. Spellings were checked and double-checked and as your daddy spelled out Frederick I looked at him one last time with that raised eyebrow, an 'Are you sure?' kind of stare. He was and we were duly packed off with your birth certificate labelled up Frederick David Jackson Bland. Our boy was official and that was the last I'd have to worry about hearing the name Frederick. I had compromised, acted like a grown-up and now I could forget all about it. Uh no. Just a couple of days later I was sat in the GP's surgery with you for one of your check-up appointments. The footsteps of the nurse clipped down the corridor followed by a loud shout for 'Frederick Bland?' The hairs on the back of my neck stood up – so much for never having to use the full version of your name. I went home for a few cross little words with Daddy.

I'd always just wanted you to be able to have Freddie on your passport and not have 'Frederick!' shouted out on the register at school. But it seemed once you had it written on a legal document it was hard to use the shortened form. After a bit of investigation I discovered that, for the more indecisive among us, you could change a baby's first name within the first twelve months of registration if another name was more regularly used. The amended name can be added into space no. 17 of the full birth certificate and this seemed perfect, as at the top it still says Frederick, keeping the rest of the family happy, but legally you can now use Freddie. This of course can easily confuse people and your first passport still arrived in the name of Frederick and had to be returned immediately for a replacement. I hope you are more decisive than your mummy, Fred, and have the courage of your convictions. If you really believe in something, be it a name or a cause, then stand your ground. I eventually got you that passport saying FREDDIE DAVID JACKSON BLAND, shortly before we had you christened Frederick. To quote one of your Grandad Hodges' one-liners again … I used to be indecisive but now I'm not so sure.

* * *

One of the early highlights of new parenthood comes in the first weeks to make up for those sleepless nights and restless evenings – baby's first smile! And your big beamer appeared out of nowhere like a lightning bolt through my heart after a feed in the lounge at five weeks old. Your gorgeous little face lit up as a big gummy grin spread across it. I tickled your chest and squeaked at you in overexcited baby talk and the smiles just kept coming. The first few weeks with a newborn you don't get a lot back, apart from the odd puke or poo. Their eyes don't really focus on you, most reactions are just reflexes and the love can very much feel all one way. But wow, as soon as you broke out the smiles that was it. As if I couldn't love you any more, suddenly my beautiful Fred could light my heart and a room at a thousand paces.

I took so many pictures and videos of that smile, it was generally agreed among all who saw them that you really were the most smiley of babies. Any little tickle or coo would elicit one of your cheeky grins and while they are currently interspersed with the odd cross-frowned toddler tantrum, your now beautiful white-toothed smile just breaks my heart with its perfect innocence and beauty. You have had a tough start in life, my Fred, having to grow up without your mummy by your side when you most need her, but I hope with all my heart that I have left enough love around you to keep that beautiful smile on your perfect little face as often as possible. When you think of me, think of love. And when you remember me always try and do it with that smile.

* * *

As with all of life there can be a competitive edge to new parenthood. The big question on everyone's lips in the early days is, 'Is your baby sleeping through the night yet?' Night-time slumber suddenly takes on a whole new beauty when it is cruelly snatched away from you every three hours or so by a wailing baby that needs feeding. There are books that tell you to follow a regimented plan to the very second. These seemed too strict to me. Then there are others that advocate attachment parenting, co-sleeping and 'wearing' your baby in a sling at all times. This seemed a bit too 'earth mother' and also not really my thing. Not having been around babies before I had no strong opinions either way, so Daddy and I fell somewhere in the middle, in the section marked 'chaos'.

From that very first night we spent together in the side room of the maternity ward, you just weren't a fan of sleeping flat on your back. You were quite a 'refluxy' baby and you basically vomited up much of the milk I'd spent the previous forty minutes or so feeding you, every time! So, I think you found it uncomfortable lying flat after a feed. Yet with all the guidelines around the terrifying sudden infant death syndrome, the advice was always that a baby should lay flat on its back in a crib with nothing else in it. It became clear this was not for you though.

The holy grail of 'the routine' evaded us. I've told you about our difficulties getting timings right when we go anywhere and it was the same with you and sleep. We never seemed to have the feed, burping, snoozing bit in the right order. There's a phenomenon some parents call 'the witching hour' where babies become unbearably fussy around five every evening. Well, you went all the way to Hogwarts and back with all-out wailing through until nine. The only way to settle you was to pop you in a sling, generally worn by Daddy, while he paced at high speed around the lounge wearing a path into the carpet. Eventually you'd snuggle into his chest and settle off into a lovely deep sleep and Daddy would then have to spend the rest of the evening trying to eat his dinner and drink his glass of wine without spilling it down the back of your neck! But he totally loved every second of those evenings with his precious boy curled up snugly on his chest. Which was lucky really because there were a lot of middle-of-the-night and early-morning chest snuggles for him as well as he battled to stay awake while trying to give me a few hours off between the night feeds.

Then there were those wild-eyed moments at 5 a.m. in our bedroom as we struggled to get you to sleep on your back in the bedside crib, where we literally would have spent a year's wages on any sort of gadget to help you sleep better. Many rash purchases were made online in the wee small hours, such as special cushions to help prop your cot up a little to aid sleep, the dream sheep that mimicked a mother's heartbeat, thin sleeping bags, thick sleeping bags … the list was endless. But none of them seemed to make much difference at all. As it turns out, sometimes in life you can't fix everything. You've just got to ride out the storm and hope it spits you out in one piece on the other side!

The Freddie-shaped night-time tornado finally spat us out onto the hallowed yellow brick road at around the twelve-week mark. This is when I happened upon a wonderful woman called Evelyn, otherwise known as 'The Cheshire Baby Whisperer', a former midwife and health visitor who knows all there is to know about babies. Her book and her replies to my endless emails hit just the right note with me. She helped us to create a routine for you and to self-settle but without ever having to leave you to 'cry it out'. Your dad and I are made of tough stuff, but not when it comes to you crying. We could never shut the door leaving you upset on the other side, which is why frequently one of us still lies next to you on the bed for an hour at a time while you go off to sleep. (This was before we broke our routine after we had to move you into a toddler bed!) So, the lovely Evelyn suggested moving you from your cramped little bedside crib into your own cot. She showed us how to get you into a routine, using soothing coloured lights and a sensory-led approach, a calming bath-time and, most importantly, no crying! Within a couple of weeks our difficult-to-settle fussy baby was dropping off like a champ. We'd literally pop you in the cot, walk out and you'd be off to sleep for the night. That gave Mummy and Daddy their all-important baby-free evenings together and a good night's sleep. Well, we would have been able to sleep if we'd just cut back a bit on technology …

I've explained how I bought pretty much every baby gadget going and as an overanxious new mum I of course wanted the top-of-the-range video baby monitor to keep a close watch on you as you slept peacefully in your cot. You were really quite an addictive watch! But along with the baby monitor came an over-the-top piece of technology called a sleep apnoea alarm. And you know sometimes a gadget can just have too many functions. Your Auntie Claire had already shaken her head wearily at our latest high-tech purchase saying, 'It'll just stress you out'. And by God that alarm was the bane of our lives. It consisted of a sensor pad which was to be placed under your mattress and hooked up to the monitor which sounded a shrill alarm if it deemed you not to have taken a breath for twenty seconds. Now if you imagine the pressure required from a skinny little four-month-old's lungs to keep some sort of sensor happy under a good three inches of mattress, you'll understand we had a bit of a reverse princess and the pea situation happening. Also, the sensor pad was tiny, so any time you rolled off it Daddy and I would be jolted awake by its incessant beeping, then have to stumble around in the dark banging heads and stubbing toes in the race to come and turn the bloody thing off before it woke you up! As soon as we had regained the energy to work out how to unhook that damn sensor pad we chucked it way into the back of the junk cupboard. A good lesson for me in life that sometimes the most expensive of something isn't necessarily the best.

* * *

Your first Christmas was a special time – both Daddy and I love the festive period. It was the first year he'd persuaded me to get a 'real' Christmas tree instead of the glittery monstrosity I'd had since living in my flat in Hale. In my head, I remembered the pine trees of my youth, with long and spindly branches that swiftly dropped their few pine needles all over the carpet, Grandma cursing them each time she had to hoover. For years I have laboured under the misapprehension that artificial trees had a better shape and were less messy. But no, thank goodness Daddy came along and we started our Bland family Christmas tradition that year of going to a little garden centre down the road in Mobberley and umming and ahhing over which was the perfect Christmas fir. Once the ideal one was picked (it would always look so much bigger when we got it home!), I'd be into the shop to buy that year's wooden decoration for it and then go about the job of persuading Daddy to buy me one of the giant stags made from twigs that were on display. We currently have three – you call them your 'heees' – horses. There is a daddy hee, a mummy hee and a baby hee. Three best friends, remember?

We always go decked out in our Christmas jumpers and woolly hats, and that first year you had an array of fabulous festive attire to choose from. I finally plumped for the furry reindeer onesie and that photo of the three of us happily preparing for our first Christmas together is one of my favourites. The other is what I will call your 'peak baby-cute' photo. Mummy's friend Auntie Dawn had bought you the most adorable little red-and-green baby elf outfit and we decided to try it out with you wearing an adult-sized 'elf ears' Christmas hat. Cue that big beaming smile of yours and our Christmas thank-you-card photo was in the bag!

We had a wonderful family day, starting by opening a few of your many presents at home with Daddy and Grandma. I'd told myself not to get too many as you really didn't know what was going on, but of course throughout December they had just piled up! We unwrapped the new bits of noisy, brightly coloured plastic junk to add to our collection and you happily slobbered away on pieces of wrapping paper. A trip to church in your obligatory Christmas jumper was followed by a lovely family afternoon at Gran and Grumpy's with Auntie Claire, Uncle Mark and the rest of the Harrison clan. Stuffed full of turkey, chocolate and wine – well, milk for you – we rolled back home to crash out in front of the TV in the traditional British style.

I do so hope that Christmas continues to be a magical time for you, my Fred. I know that Father Christmas (*never* Santa Claus – we are NOT American!) will be extra kind to you. If that first Christmas together with you and all the Blands, Hodges and Harrisons taught me anything, it's that there is an incredible amount of love around us in this family. I hope you carry on the tradition of going to get that beautiful tree from Mobberley, and every year get a new decoration, a really sparkly beautiful one, and hang it on there from me. I'm so sorry that I can't be there to watch you open your gifts myself, but I hope I have left behind enough of my most precious gift of all. A mother's never-ending love.

* * *

I adored being a new mum and soon got into the swing of packing up half the house every time I wanted to go somewhere with you. Babies require a lot of paraphernalia even just to pop out for a coffee with friends. Spare nappies, wipes, changes of clothes (for both you and Mummy in case that reflux vomit headed my way!), Sudocrem, muslin cloths, breastfeeding cover scarf, pointless toys to wave at you, later a Sophie giraffe to chew on while you were teething, dribble bibs …

I could go on and on and that's before you've even got the pram and car seat in the car. Leaving the house really was a military-style operation.

I loved being on maternity leave either at home with you or meeting up with my new mummy friends from the NCT group for coffee and cake or my friends from work who had had babies around the same time. Cute little babies like you were, Fred, can be quite demanding in terms of the number of times they need something in the day – you fed around every three hours for about forty minutes. I recorded all this along with your nap times religiously in a baby-tracking app on my phone. For a while there I think I got a little too into making pretty routine patterns in the graphs it would provide!

After the early days of struggling to get you to latch on properly and feed enough, things finally began to settle down. It turned out that you had something called 'tongue-tie' where the little string of tissue that attaches the tongue to the bottom of the mouth is too short and can restrict movement and make feeding more difficult. It can in some cases affect speech in later life and it runs in families. I know this because once they'd said you had it I looked under my own tongue and lo and behold, I had exactly the same! I checked in with Grandma and it would seem that back in the days when Mummy was born they weren't as bothered about it because Grandma couldn't remember it ever being mentioned. It obviously didn't affect my speech, as look what I ended up doing, but it does explain why I always looked ridiculous if I tried to poke my tongue out in a photo as a teenager. (The 'poking tongue out' pose makes everyone look slightly odd, I think – that's definitely one to be avoided.) These days, though, midwives are immediately on the lookout for it as it can be very simply fixed with a small snip using a teeny pair of scissors while a baby is still tiny. This is done by a trained nurse, by the way. Mummy wasn't about to come at you with a little pair of nail scissors! They promised no blood and no pain, though it sounded terrifying to me.

Despite it being such a quick procedure we still had to wait eight weeks for our good old NHS appointment, at which point you seemed much more alert and aware of what was happening. Not for the last time I had to let Daddy hold you to have it done while I cowered in the corner of the room, covering my ears and praying you weren't feeling any pain. I was much the same with all your injections and really any time you fell over. I just can't bear for my little boy to suffer in any way. Of course as soon as the tongue-tie was snipped I swooped straight in and cuddled you close. At least it was done now and we could move onwards, feeding you up into the strong little boy you've become.

The only slight issue was that feeding was going TOO well. Now we had got the hang of it, your weight was progressing in the right direction, you fed quickly and with decent long gaps in between. I was able to express loads of extra milk (we had a freezer full of the stuff) in the hope that Daddy could give you a bottle or two each day to both bond with you, as dads don't get much of a look-in in the first months, and also to give me a break and the ability to go out on my own if I wanted to. But this was the moment we began to get an inkling of your incredibly stubborn nature, which you have inherited directly from me. It's a Hodges family trait. When we decide we do or don't want to do something we have an unbending will of iron and nothing can knock us off our path. Right now, if you decide you are unhappy about something and you don't want to do it, your cross face and grunts of 'NO! I DON'T LIKE' would have even the most evil of dictators thinking twice about crossing you. I feel on the whole this is a positive thing, as I've talked already about having the courage of your convictions. You might just have to be aware that those around you will still be hoping for a bit of compromise!

In the early days of breastfeeding you're advised not to introduce a bottle so as not to confuse the baby. We duly waited until you were six weeks old and all seemed to be going swimmingly. Daddy would get home from work and give you your last feed of expressed milk in a bottle before we 'tried' putting you to bed. This was pre-baby whisperer! Daddy loved his bonding time with you and being able to take an active role in growing his son. Then he had a particularly busy time and a week went by without him doing it. We thought nothing of it and the next time he was around we heated up your little bottle to the perfect warm temperature, but as Daddy held you in his arms you turned your gorgeous little face away from that bottle and point-blank refused to drink it. This was the start of a war that raged for the next six months … We called it the 'Blands' Bottle Battle' and it was brutal.

We sought advice online, from friends and from health visitors. 'How can we get our baby to take a bottle?' was searched a thousand times on Google. The health visitor told me it was obviously because I was doing such a good job of feeding you myself – oh, she knew how to get me on side! But it became the most frustrating issue in your first year. The general advice seemed to be to keep trying, so every day we'd defrost some milk, heat it up and end up pouring it down the sink while muttering quiet profanities under our breath as you resolutely stayed a baby-bottle refusenik. The other suggestion was to 'try different brands of bottle'. Oooh, an opportunity to buy more things! But the kitchen cupboards slowly filled up with an array of baby bottles, all tried and refused.

Every once in a while you would randomly nail a whole bottle. Just to show us you could if you wanted to. We'd try not to get too excited while it was happening and scare you off the precious bottle, so we'd be grinning at each other and hitting silent high-fives. We'd send a celebratory WhatsApp message to our NCT gang, some of whom had been having similar issues. But soon we learnt this was premature. One day you'd down 150 ml from a bottle like you'd emerged from days in the Sahara, the next you'd turn your head away from it and keep that little mouth of yours firmly shut. Even more frustrating, as you grew and your movements developed you'd just bat it away with your hands! But remember I told you that you got your will of iron from your mummy, and so I persisted. Every day I would try, holding my nerve, internalizing the worst of the swear words as I poured unused milk away. And suddenly, after eight long months of you being solely breastfed, and by then partly weaned, you deigned to start drinking from the bottle. The wonderful irony was that as you grew into a toddler you then refused to have bedtime milk from anything else. The advice is to start using a sippy cup from the age of one so the milk doesn't pool behind a baby's teeth and cause tooth decay. But you would hand anything back that wasn't in one of your precious bottles until you stopped having bedtime milk just before you were three. Yeah, perhaps Mummy didn't win on that after all!

* * *

I've talked about my love of a neutral decor and having everything in its place, and before we had you I had grand plans for the house to stay looking like it did and not filling up with gaudy baby stuff. In the early days, when I had a choice I'd always pick the toys, chairs and teddies in lovely tones of grey, brown, cream and white. Auntie Claire laughed at me knowingly. Just you wait she said, the bright colours will come. And they did. It turned out while baby's sight is developing bright colours are the thing. Everything comes in lurid shades of durable plastic and wipe-clean material. Pretty soon our lounge looked like a particularly unwell unicorn had come along and vomited a rainbow of colours over everything we owned. And the noise!? Every developmental baby toy has to come with some sort of tinny, loud, overly fast nursery rhymes that just keep playing on repeat. Every night, as I'd try to drop off to sleep, those damn baby songs would just keep playing in my head. When you catch yourself humming them while you're out and about you know you're in trouble. They're enough to drive you to the asylum!

Chief offender among the plastic, brightly coloured, noisy baby toys was the fabled 'Jumperoo'. It is a rite of passage that every baby must bounce in one for at least half of their first six months. It's a plastic circle – yours was covered in red, green, blue and yellow safari animals – and you could sit in the little webbed seat in the middle and just bounce. And bounce you did, like our very own little Tigger. You would while away huge chunks of time in there, every bounce rattling the thing like mad and shaking the house to its very foundations. You practically wore a hole in the carpet with your enthusiasm. I think it must be where you get your strong climbing legs from now. You would happily stomp along in that chair to the strains of 'Froggy Went a Courting', and despite it taking up a lot of space in the lounge, and not blending in with the colour scheme in any way, I loved that Jumperoo. You were happy, and it gave me a few minutes to sit down with a coffee in front of some rubbishy daytime TV. This was of course before you became the one true holder of the TV controller.

* * *

Apart from the 'Blands' Bottle Battle', the other main thing I stressed about when you were growing up in the first year were the 'baby milestones'. These are developmental moments that show a baby is progressing normally and there are lists online of the age ranges by which certain skills should be reached. Again it played into the competitive nature in me as other mums compared timings of when their babies had reached each one. Among the first biggies was rolling over, a sign that your core strength was improving and you were developing the muscles to get crawling. A good way to help baby reach this milestone was 'tummy time', popping you onto your tummy on a mat with toys and books in front of you to amuse you. Problem was, with your reflux, every time I put you on your tummy you'd immediately vomit, so I decided we could probably get through without! So it took a little while for you to roll over – at about four months as I recall – but as ever, when you decide to do something you really do it well. I'd popped you on your big cushioned mat at the end of the room and, expecting you to stay where I left you as normal, I went into the kitchen to make a cup of tea. When I returned, my heart dropped to the floor for a second, as I clocked a completely empty mat, no Freddie to be seen! A few hurried steps further into the lounge and I caught sight of you, a good seven feet away from where I'd left you, playing with the long cord of the blinds. I of course stopped to snap a quick picture to send to Daddy, before disentangling you and noting that we now needed to start 'baby-proofing' the house. Even from just a few months old, my Freddie, you've been able to do anything you set your mind to. You just need to keep on rolling to where you want to go in life and you'll be just fine.

* * *

It was around this time of you barrel-rolling around the house that it was decided something had to be done about 'the hair'. I told you how you were born with that thick dark mop of hair. In most babies it gradually falls out over the first few months as new hair grows through. Yours sort of did a bit of what Grandad Hodges would have called a 'botch-job'. Where you lay on your back in your cot at night you'd turn your little head from side to side, as babies do, which would rub away lots of those little early baby locks. But only around the widest part of your head. It led to the first of your hairstyles we named affectionately 'the reverse monk'. You had a big circle of dark hair on top, were totally bald around the middle, and then had more long dark hair at the bottom, which kept on growing longer and longer, mullet-style! This was later followed by 'the Lloyd', when you had your first proper haircut and the way the hairdresser cut your fringe short and straight across made you look a little like the characters in another top-notch movie, *Dumb and Dumber*. My favourite, though, was always when it was long enough to get in a little topknot! This was only ever done at the hands of your cousins Imogen and Matilda, and would always signal the 'he needs a haircut' look from Daddy!

You have such beautiful hair. It's something people have always commented on and has always made you look older than you are. You know what I'm going to say here don't you …? Yep, you get it from Mummy's side! I'm claiming all the good bits. People always tell me I have thick hair, though technically it's not. It's fairly fine but there is a LOT of it. It comes from the Hodges side of the family and Grandad Hodges' dad, my grandfather, had a full head of thick hair when he died in his eighties. Your Uncle Matthew is the same, past forty and no signs of a bald patch. I'm not sure what happened to poor old Grandad Hodges, as his started going thin in his twenties, earning him the nickname 'Fluff'!

Your hair is one of the things I have put into the hands of your Auntie Claire and told her to keep it 'Boden-model long' for as long as you'll allow. When you're old enough you will make your own decisions about what to do with it, I guess, but until then I'm keeping control from wherever I am! But speaking of control, I had none over 'the reverse monk'. The middle bit kept getting more and more bald, but above and below it kept growing longer and longer. A good three inches of dark hair hung down the back of your neck. There were repeated suggestions from Grandma to perhaps just 'give it a snip', but I kept reading things online about how you shouldn't cut a baby's hair in the first year as it could damage it. Things came to a head, literally, one Saturday at your swimming lesson. We used to take you every week, to the very expensive and wholly pointless classes that involved Daddy mostly standing around in warm water waiting for his turn to dunk you under. I was watching from the side, snapping away pictures on my phone as I normally do, when you emerged from a dip under the water with all that dark hair plastered down your face and neck. I suddenly had an epiphany moment that it really looked quite odd next to the other fairly bald babies in the pool. I relented and got out a very teeny blunt pair of scissors at home and spent the next few days gradually snipping it into something resembling normal. 'The reverse monk' was no more.

* * *

Another big milestone moment from the first year of babyhood is the process of weaning. It's a long and complicated mission of introducing solid foods for the first time alongside your milk. I was a goody-two-shoes and followed the health visitor's advice to the letter – waiting until you were six months old and your little tummy was well developed. However, as I've already said, I am no domestic goddess. Cooking is very much your dad's thing, but I did my best to turn Stepford Wife while weaning and got busy whipping up purées of every kind of vegetable and fruit imaginable. The idea is to get a baby used to lots of different tastes so they have a good palate in later life. Well, obviously I didn't do that great a job as at the moment, if we were to let you exist solely on chips, peas, strawberries and pasta, then that's what you would do!

Weaning was a messy affair and there seemed to be so many vegetables involved that were bright orange, an impossible stain to get out of your clothes and mine, where it would invariably end up. We went through packs and packs of baby wipes. Food got in your eyes, hair, ears, on the tray, on the floor. I swiftly moved from small bibs onto the long-sleeved smock affairs. I once considered just stripping you down to a nappy before mealtimes to save on washing. I even thought of my *Dragons' Den* business idea: full boiler suits for weaning parents, which save on the washing when your baby sneezes on a spoonful of butternut-squash purée! I also pondered whether porridge needed a rebrand as superglue – seriously, next time you smash an ornament just stick it back together with some of the oaty stuff! You once spent a full day with a porridge-smeared eyebrow. Despite repeated attempts there was no way to get it off until bath-time.

Alongside the many purées, an important part of the weaning process is allowing babies to learn how to feed themselves by providing them with finger foods. You used to love chewing away on chunks of pitta bread, fingers of banana and apricot pieces. Often, though, you would literally bite off more than you could chew. This was swiftly followed by the initiation of your gag reflex and a good old baby vomit. Not a problem at the start of a meal. Very much a problem the time I'd just fed you a lurid green purée while you wore a cream top and trousers. You live and learn.

* * *

When you were nearly nine months old we introduced you to another Bland family tradition, our annual summertime trip to Salcombe. This is another one of our happy places that I know Daddy will continue to take you to as you grow. Salcombe Harbour is a little slice of heaven in Devon. We started visiting there on our first wedding anniversary and have been every year since. As I'm sure you'll know by now, Daddy is very much a sea-faring fellow having taught windsurfing for a number of seasons in his youth. He is one of those people who is always happy just messing about on boats and taking to the water. He's really missed being by the coast since he moved back up north from Southampton, leaving all his windsurfing rig far behind, so it lifts his soul to be back by the sea. And if Daddy is happy, then I am happy. I've always loved the coast and harboured, if you'll excuse the pun, dreams of retiring down to Salcombe one day. I had such lovely visions of us all spending the summers of our future there in a beautiful, big house overlooking the estuary. Sandy shoes cast off by the door, glasses of wine being drunk, while the day's events on the beach or water are dissected with laughter. I would look over at you, my beautiful son, so proud of the growing man you will one day become, for I know whatever may come I will always be proud of you, Freddie.

You approach Salcombe from high up on the hill and get your first glimpse of the sea to the right over the rolling-green fields. Then, as the road dips down into town, there are the most stunning views across the estuary to the golden sandy beaches of East Portlemouth, a two-minute ferry ride across from the steps at the bottom of the Ferry Inn. The main narrow street through Salcombe is one-way, so you loop through town to head up the hill. And it's just the kind of street where Mummy can do a lot of damage, with all my favourite brands just lined up, one after the other! We always take an early trip down there shopping to grab a few new items of nautical-inspired clothing to wear during our stay. It's the home of Jack Wills clothing, one of Mummy's favourites. I always think it's rude not to buy some merch while in its home town. And of course there are plenty of ice-cream stops to keep little boys happy. It was on this trip that you had your first taste of ice cream, as Daddy carried you in the backpack. Incredibly for a boy who will now polish off ice creams like they're his last meal, you weren't too convinced. A little too cold, I think, judging by the faces you were pulling!

At the bottom of the hill is the famous Cranch's Sweet Shop with its iconic pink-and-white candy-striped awning. And beyond that the road snakes around to various art galleries – we always have to buy some Salcombe-inspired art on each trip as well, something I hope you'll help Daddy with choosing in the future. Then the harbour wall stretches across in front of you, a great spot for a bit of crabbing as you gaze out at the boats bobbing around on the harbour and, of course, your favourite thing from this year's trip – the RNLI lifeboat. Real-life Fireman Sam stuff – it totally blew your mind!

Over the years we've stayed in all sorts of places, with the only downside being that most involved steps, and Daddy had to lug your junk up and down them. But this first trip we'd played a blinder and found the lovely Cliff Cottage, a beautiful yellow end-of-terrace right next to the yacht club. Even though the holiday cottage was advertised as family-friendly, we still had to do a bit of furniture rearranging as you were crawling and cruising around everywhere and grabbing everything you could. You made a beeline for the very funky coffee table made out of various (and sharp!) iron tools, so that was tucked away behind the sofas. A metal fire poker you took a shine to had to be hidden in the games chest and all the precious-looking ornaments moved to a much higher level. We weren't about to lose our deposit!

Grandma came down to join us for a few days and it was a wonderful first family holiday. We did all the things that make up our perfect trips to Salcombe. A bit of beach time, lunch at The Winking Prawn, dinner at the Victoria Inn. You were at that halcyon age where we could get you to sleep in your pram and head out for dinner with you fast asleep and have a proper evening out. Quite the opposite to this year where, despite staying in the luxury of the Salcombe Harbour Hotel, dinners were taken early and mostly alone by me, as Daddy chased you around the decking outside!

The last couple of years we have been blessed with the most incredible weather on our trips there. I always say that standing on the golden sandy beach at East Portlemouth, looking towards the pretty pastel cottages of Salcombe across the estuary, with the sun glinting off the water and fabulous yachts cruising in and out of the harbour, you really could be in the south of France. But without having to wrestle you into submission on a two-hour flight to get there. I can tell how much you already love it there, as this year you spent so much time on the balcony of our room excitedly pointing out 'pirate ships' and 'fishing boats' and Fireman Sam's 'Neptune' boat. We have made some wonderful memories in that happy little town, Freddie, and I hope you and your daddy make many more. It is one of the places I urge you to go to when you want to picture me at my most content and feel my spirit around you.

* * *

Suddenly, in the merest blink of an eye, my teeny-tiny snuggly little newborn was one. When you're juggling a wailing baby on your knee with dark-ringed eyes from the sleep deprivation, there is always a kindly older lady nearby who smiles and says, 'Ah, enjoy it while you can, they're not little for long'. I, like most fraught new mothers, would quietly resist the urge to slap them while smiling through gritted teeth. But you know what, they were right. You were now almost a toddler, not quite walking yet, but nearly. Your first birthday party called for an actual pair of shoes – some funky navy Converse. Prior to this you lived in socks, or generally bare feet as socks stayed on but for a moment with the speed at which you were crawling around.

The first birthday party is a rite of passage and I was determined to do a top job of it for you, my Fred. This obviously involved a lot of work ... for Grumpy! Having ripped out most of the garden at the start of the summer, it was a race against time to get it looking perfect for your party in September. This involved some of the following tasks – fencing, grass relaying, border planting, decking building and the pièce de résistance, your first birthday present of a climbing-frame fort complete with swings! Wow, he was glad you only turned one once. It all got finished, literally on the morning of the party, then he and Daddy were despatched to buy the perfect potted tree for the new decking. I'm nothing if not a perfectionist! Our lovely new garden sofa was in place and 'HAPPY 1ST BIRTHDAY' banners were strung up on the fences. We rented a load of soft-play kit which was laid out on the lawn, perfect for you and your little crawling buddies to bump around on.

We had the most lovely afternoon with you, all our friends and your little playmates. The sun shone and people were even nice about the cake I made. They may have spat it out into their napkins with their next breath, but at the very least it looked fabulous. I toiled over that cake for you, Freddie – the first I had ever made! Just like I'm not much of a cook, I am not much of a baker. But I had practised and got tips from all the pros. My attempts were hampered somewhat by our ancient old cooker that only seems to have one setting which is 'fire of Hades'. But once you've cut the more blackened bits off, then no one is any the wiser. It was safari-themed so I had decided to cover it in green fondant icing I would roll out myself, as well as some yellow 'safari-style grass' around the bottom, and I had bought some 'safari animal' cake toppers and your name written in icing from a way more talented lady on eBay. Of course I had also bought as much cake-baking kit as possible to make all this happen! Baking tins, parchment, paintbrushes, cake glue, rolling pins, icing smoothers – I was channelling Mary Berry like a pro! (You may have to look her up.) But of course all the gear, no idea. Despite a successful attempt at icing a practice cake, when it came to the big moment I think I over-rolled the fondant and as I tried to pick it up with the rolling pin, as I had successfully done once before, it began to crack and dropped back onto the work surface in two torn pieces. I think my shouts of frustration were heard all the way into town and they definitely brought Daddy sprinting in from the garden. After a bit of deep breathing and a bit of sticking back together, the cake was rescued, icing smoothed (with my new cake smoothers!) and you know what? When it was finished I was pretty chuffed with it. It may have tasted like a rock but it looked good, and sometimes in life it's okay to go with a bit of style over substance, Fred, as long as you don't make a habit of it.

The photo that was taken of you, Daddy and I happily cuddled together in the garden on that afternoon remains one of my favourite and most happy memories, when life was still innocent and full of hope for our future as a family. I made it my Facebook profile picture and have never changed it and never will now as I love that jofyul snapshot in time. It was just a few weeks later that I found the lump that would change the course of all our lives forever. We will come back to that moment later. But for now let's savour that happy family snapshot of us Blands. The three best friends that anyone could have.

Chapter 9

FROM BOUNCING BABY TO MY BEAUTIFUL BOY

In the months leading up to your first birthday you had been getting around the house at the pace of Red Rum. You started crawling early at seven months. I would pop you down in the lounge, walk into the kitchen to get something and literally trip over you as you appeared at a rate of knots on all fours behind me. This progressed to you pulling yourself up to a standing position using any nearby piece of furniture, person or often by grabbing tufts of fur on poor old Bodie. Then 'cruising' around the house, using those same props to help you walk about. The downstairs part of the house was quickly baby-proofed until there was basically nothing below a metre from the floor in our lounge. Many of the framed photos and ornaments that we packed away remain gathering dust in the garage, never to see the light of day again. I thought you'd be an early walker, but as your first birthday came and went you just didn't want to quite let go of the stabilizers! Then, just as I was about to get myself worked up into a baby-milestone-missed frenzy, two weeks after your first birthday party you took us by surprise with your most adorable first steps. And as luck would have it both Daddy and I were there to experience the wonderful moment together.

You had been doing your usual cruising around the sofas early one evening when suddenly you just went hell for leather across the living room, arms held aloft, your little hips wiggling and a look of pure joy on your little face as you practically ran across the room. This was met with much squealing – me – and cheering – Dad – and you warmed to your audience. Every time you lost your balance you'd touch your hands down to the floor then swing them back up high and carry on staggering around like a drunken baby orangutan. We of course captured the big moment on video to proudly send around to all the family. Just thinking about it now makes my heart swell with love and happiness at the sparkle in your eye and your own personal elation at making your first steps in this world. From this moment there would be no stopping you on your journey through this life.

* * *

I've mentioned the wonderful Bodie so many times, but it bears repeating what an absolute hero of a dog he is. I grew up with golden retrievers as a child and knew they were such a gentle and loving breed of dog. When we had first got Bodie after just nine months together, it had been very much with a view that he would be the dog our children would grow up around. We got him from a breeder in Carmarthen – a nice Welsh boy he is – and we met his mum, Isa, when we went to visit him as a tiny snuggly puppy. She was such a dainty and gentle retriever, he obviously inherited her sweet nature and his father's stunningly regal good looks. The breeder also told us the father had a super temperament. We followed all the puppy guidance to the letter, took him to his training classes and were well rewarded, as he grew into a dog I can confidently say to be the most sensitive, gentle and loving animal I have ever had the luck to meet. He had just over two years of being our number-one furry son before you came along to usurp his position at the top of our affections. He always remained only a hair's breadth in second, though!

In those two years he was the apple of our eye. I guess he was our practice go at being parents. There were night-time wakings in the early days, another life you had to think about before yours. Some people may scoff at the idea, but I really think having a dog prepares you in some small way for parenthood. All our time was spent out walking with Bodie in Tatton Park, Alderley Edge and Lyme Park. He is never happier than when he is running free and chasing a ball. We uploaded so many pictures of our beautiful golden boy to Facebook it became a running joke, and every time we saw our friend Paul, he'd sarcastically say 'Wow, have you got a dog? I didn't know!'

As you would expect, Bodie took your arrival in his stride and soon got used to the new member of the family. As you grew and began to move around, you would alternately use him as a pillow, a walking aid and a playmate. We would referee the two of you as best we could to make sure you weren't hurting him or pulling his furry tail too much, but he tolerated pretty much everything you could throw at him. And I mean that literally. Just this morning a 'memory video' appeared on my social media of him lying down as you crawl on his back, gently banging him with a squishy ball that makes a very irritating 'BOIIIINGGG!' noise. And he just lies there, looking up at us with his big, beautiful, brown eyes as if to say 'Am I doing okay here? Mummy, is this right?' Never did he snap, growl, snarl or even curl a lip at you. He rarely even got up and walked away from your relentless cuddly assaults. The two of you formed a wonderful bond and I love to see how much you adore him as you throw your arms around his neck and tell him 'I love you so much, Bodie'.

Your dad and I are very much country folk and we love stomping around fields in our flat caps, Barbour jackets and wellies. Come rain or shine we would be out and about with you and Bodie. I used to love our walks with you, me and Bodie in Tatton Park while I was on maternity leave. I'd put you in the baby carrier on my back and we'd head into Dog Wood together and take Bodie for a swim in Tatton Mere. Those were some of my most confident moments of motherhood; I felt strong as I strode along, taking my two boys out. Once your walking was a little more proficient than 'drunken orangutan baby' we often took Bodie to the woods behind Beggarman's Lane, as it was a much shorter distance for your little wobbly legs to toddle. I would spend a lot of the time picking you up and dusting your hands down as you tripped over various sticks and tree roots or just over your own ridiculously cute first tiny pair of blue-and-red wellies. As you got more steady on your feet you began to insist on holding the 'wah', what we sniggeringly called 'the wanger', which was a plastic ball-throwing contraption used to hurl tennis balls for miles for Bodie to chase. Unfortunately, your desire to hold the 'wah' did not match up with your motor skills at that time, so poor Bodie spent a lot of time eyeing it longingly as you waggled it around, unable to release the tennis ball from the end. He would sometimes lose patience and just grab the ball out of it and run away with his prize. But you didn't mind as long as you held onto 'wah'. Much like the fabled TV controller, he who holds the wanger holds the power.

* * *

You love your freedom, much preferring those walks in the woods to the many baby and toddler classes I paid fortunes to take you to that were generally swiftly dropped after a term. I always say you are NOT a fan of organized fun. All the other toddlers at Rhythm Time, Tumble Tots and toddler group would happily sit in a circle singing along and doing actions to the songs, while I would spend the whole time chasing you around the room trying to stop you playing with the plug sockets or pulling out forbidden bits of apparatus and attempting to stop it from turning into a fun game of chase! You have so much energy and a free spirit and I wouldn't have it any other way. If you were ever frowned upon, that would be the point when I'd decide that class probably wasn't the one for us. I think it's that determined mind of yours you are showing already, but you much prefer to set the agenda when it comes to your own playtime. You are most happy meeting up with your little NCT playmates at the ice-cream farm down the road. Unlike most of the other children you sprint past the ice-cream counter and out into the playground, dashing around from sandpit to play-car to swing like you're on a toddler version of *Total Wipeout*. Sometimes it's hard to keep track of you while I'm trying to chat to my friends and there'll be a heart-stopping moment where I lose sight of you and panic. Then I spot your little head whizzing past the window, hair bouncing as you make a beeline for your favourite motorbike one of the other children has just finished with.

Sometimes I do manage to get you inside to eat an ice cream and what a tense experience that is, only to be attempted with the steadiest of nerves. You are a very slow eater just like your mummy and Grandad Hodges before her. Not a great combination with a fast-melting foodstuff. Add to that your tendency to then start eating the cone from the bottom up with most of the ice cream still on the top, so I spend much of the time like an octopus with wipes trying to catch the drips and a few of my anguished tears!

Then you'll get fed up, dump the ice cream on the tray and get back to another of your favourite pastimes while there: driving the long-suffering owner round the bend by pushing little plastic stools up and down the floor with your mate Darcy, making the most irritating scraping noise known to man. Do I sound like an irresponsible mother here, my Fred? Because I'm really not. It just gives me joy to see you doing things that give *you* joy, and hey, if that means everyone listening to some ear-splitting stool-pushing for a couple of minutes, then I'm down with that. I do draw the line somewhere though, and the time you lobbed a cup of water over one of the sofas, then got caught by the boss-lady pulling the safety padding off one of the interior pillars, you were reprimanded and packed off home before you got us all banned from there for ever.

* * *

Not long after you started walking you went through a stage of insisting on staying in the car after every journey and having a 'drive'. One of us would sit in the front with you, having a bit of quiet 'parent phone time', while you would stand on the front seat grabbing the steering wheel for all you were worth like Lewis Hamilton wrestling his Mercedes around Eau Rouge. Your eyes would sparkle with delight as you rather aggressively waggled the indicator levers and switched the hazard-warning lights on and off. Sometimes we'd have to step in and stop you posting old coins and parking receipts into the air vents. But many happy hours were whiled away on the driveway. Who needs those cheap plastic kids' cars when your toddler can have so much fun in the expensive full-sized version? Well, more fool Mummy and Daddy when we discovered that pressing the central-locking button on and off approximately a gazillion times in one minute is not the best way to keep it in tip-top shape. Who knew! It's especially bad if you don't notice for quite some time that the driver's side door no longer locks when you press the key fob. And worse if within that time your sat-nav screen mysteriously goes missing, never to be seen again. But what's a £350 navigation system between friends when our boy was learning and exploring his surroundings?

* * *

While you enjoy your thrill-seeking when you are in control, you have so far shown yourself not to be a 'fan of the fair'. Every year on the first weekend of May in Knutsford we have the big 'Knutsford May Day' parade and fair. It's a tradition that goes back generations. The costumes remain the same. Well, I trust they have been replaced multiple times over the years or they'd be pretty smelly by the time you get to go on a procession through town that includes marching bands, morris dancers, draught horses and men riding quite frankly dangerous-looking penny-farthing bikes. It is delightfully middle England. Your dad loves to reminisce about the year he was a clown and got so completely soaked by the lovely northern rain that his clown paint dripped down his face. But it is a Knutsford rite of passage and one we had already started speculating on: 'I wonder which costume Freddie will wear'. I so wish that I could be there, Freddie, proudly waving at my boy as you walk past in your first parade grinning at your family, or perhaps in a bit of a mood because it is organized fun after all! But know that I have pictured it in my mind's eye already, a snapshot of the future.

Once the parade has finished all the parents and children head for the funfair on the heath and so far you have not been keen. It is a kaleidoscope of colour, with flashing lights on fairground rides whirling up into the air as the older children riding them shriek with delight. Everything is packed in tightly and there are the smells of food stalls, selling anaemic-looking fairground burgers and big bags of candy floss. I probably shouldn't tell you this but the bags of candy floss are Mummy's favourites! I only have a little bit of that once a year at the fair, as it is literally spun sugar that will rot your teeth as soon as you look at it, but I love the pretty pastel colours, that weird spongy texture and how it dissolves into nothing but sweet goodness in your mouth. Just don't make a habit of eating it or you'll have bankrupted Daddy with dentist fees by the time you're a teenager.

Added to the smells, the sounds and the lights are half of Knutsford's parents pushing buggies and often with dogs in tow (we had to stop taking Bodie as he'd just keep wolfing down all the leftover food that had been dropped on the floor), and even for Mummy it's a pretty overwhelming scene. For you being fairly sensitive to all of the above it was almost too much. Year one when you were a baby you mostly buried your head into Daddy's shoulder. Year two we had high hopes for getting you on a ride with your cousins, but spent most of the time plonking you in brightly coloured plastic cars on the toddler merry-go-rounds, then having to take our lives in our hands to whip you off again as you began to shout 'I DON'T LIKE!' as they started to spin. Year three this year and we made some progress – we actually managed to splurge a nicely unreasonable amount of cash on a few rides as you went round with your friend Darcy, but your face could at best be described as unsmiling next to her look of pure joy. There was one panicky moment where you decided to shout 'I WANT TO GET OFF!' while on an inflatable spinning boat in the middle of a big inflatable pool, while the attendant was NOT paying attention, but after a bit of shouting we managed to get you off with all three of us staying dry.

With these small increments of improvement in your fair enjoyment I had hoped next year was going to be the one when we hit the jackpot and you 'got' the fun in funfair. Though I won't be here to see it, I know Daddy and all the family will. Like I've said before, you're definitely showing all the signs of being a bit more sensitive like your mummy. Sometimes we find big, loud situations in life harder to deal with. My ethos has always been that you've got to keep trying them and challenging yourself, because you get a wonderful sense of achievement when you've conquered a fear. By the way, my favourite ride at the funfair has always been the waltzer. I love the feeling of being spun around, gripping onto the bar for dear life until your neck feels like it's going to break! It makes me a bit delirious and I can't wipe the smile off my face the whole time. But none of the Bland-Harrisons like the sensation of spinning and the mere thought of it makes your dad nauseous. I had hoped you'd grow up to be my waltzer buddy and I still think you may, the amount of time you spending spinning in circles at home until you fall down dizzy. And waltzer buddies are for life.

* * *

Your moods, which I have referred to throughout this last chapter or so, are just like mine. I'm afraid you've inherited a slight bit of the Hodges' bad temper. The fact I am likening my own moods to that of a toddler is a bit of a worry, isn't it Fred, but I guess some of us are just destined to be the Peter Pans of this world! Poor Daddy is well aware of the fact that when I get in a mood about something there is just no getting me out of it until I'm good and ready. It's a very odd feeling, and perhaps one you will still recognize in yourself, but nothing anyone says or does can shake that dark cloud away until suddenly, be it five minutes or five hours later, something will just switch in my brain and

I'll forget about why I was ever angry in the first place! And this is something I see you doing all the time, but in a much cuter way than Mummy ever could. When you get cross, whether about not being able to take your battery-operated pirate ship into the bath or being offered the wrong type of snack, for the next half an hour or so the answer to everything will be a curt 'NO!', usually delivered with arms folded and brow furrowed. Your daddy always says he really regrets ever teaching you the word 'no' as we've heard it so much. I'm not sure we did teach it to you. I think it was a bit of stubbornness that was inbuilt in you from the start! But then, as if a magic wand is waved, you'll suddenly be distracted by one of your toys or TV programmes and your mood miraculously disappears.

It's so funny to see my own temperament reflected back in the toddler mirror and sometimes it makes me feel incredibly childish. But it still won't stop me from getting in a mood again the next time – though I should point out your father and I rarely have a cross word as we're both too easy-going. But here I can offer no advice on how to shorten the length of these grumpy spells. After forty years of pondering I still haven't found the answer to just snapping out of it! Sometimes in life, Freddie, there will be things you do and facets of your personality that you just can't explain or reason with. And that's okay. Just try and be aware of them and recognize them, and that's half the battle. Your daddy has a much better approach that I urge you to take on board. When we do something wrong, or have a cross word, then we just need to say sorry and everything is okay again. So simple and so easy, and one of the many reasons your daddy is the best man I have ever known.

You also take after me when it comes to getting presents and new things! We've been buying you quite a lot of stuff recently, I guess to try and ease our consciences about everything that's been happening around you. Your speech is now so good you ask for the specific toys you want. Just in the last few days that has been a 'bull do-dozer' and a 'blue crane'. I dutifully track these gifts down on Amazon for you and then have to try and explain the concept of waiting for them to arrive. You've not quite got it yet, as every time I promise you that I have got you what you've asked for you'll still cry because it's not here RIGHT NOW. But when a parcel does get delivered (by Postman Pat, obviously!) you immediately think it's for you (you are often correct in this assumption, but there are just as many for Mummy too – always a disappointing moment for you!). It's usually greeted with an 'Ooooh, a parcel. For me?' and whenever we ask you what you think is inside it you guess the wrong thing, which is a worrying moment, as you've forgotten what you've asked for! Then you get all excited, shifting from foot to foot, as we open the box. This is very much like Mummy when she's got a new handbag or some clothes in the post or a lovely present from Daddy. As I've said, I can be very childlike at times. With a smile on your face and hands clasped in delight you are always thrilled with whatever is inside, and this morning it was the blue crane. Then before we can get it out of the box, which always drives your dad and me insane as it's like some sort of Crystal Maze game to unlock it from the packaging, you start scanning the pictures on the side of the box of other toys in the range and asking for them too!

We may be spoiling you with a few too many things at the moment, but I want to be able to see that little shuffle-footed happy dance, watch your face light up as the box is opened and see the pleasure you get from playing with your new toy as often as possible for as long as I am still here. Your joy brings me joy and that is what gets me through the tough times.

You go through phases with toys and we've never pushed you into a gender-stereotyped toy choice, but you LOVE a fancy vehicle. Be it tractors, lorries, diggers, planes and trains, you have boxes full of them all. You are also quite into little figures, be it Fireman Sam or the Octonauts. In fact you like anything little, which can make life hard sometimes when you drop things while we are out or lose them at home, and Daddy and I end up crawling around on all fours looking under sofas and tables for the tiny pitchfork that you just HAVE to have at that very moment! The pitchfork came with a horse we bought you. You have a lot of horses which is probably down to Mummy. Because I love horses and riding (more of which later) I think I've always pointed them out in your books and made a big fuss about them. So in the early days 'heees', as you started off calling them, became a favourite and now any time we see a 'horsey' toy then you want it.

I hope you continue to love horses as you grow up, whether you want to ride them or not. I've not managed to get you on one yet. We were at the Bolesworth International Horse Show recently and they had little ponies doing rides around a very small enclosed ring. 'Bingo!' I thought. Here's my chance to get Freddie on a pony, as these look just his size and not too intimidating. So I took you into the little ring to see them, and you patted one as I held you. Softly, softly, catchee monkey. I tentatively asked you if you would like to get on one, but was met with a very polite, 'No, thank you'. Damn it, my grand plans to get you horse riding early scuppered again. Not one to take no for an answer, I continued to ask you all the time we were there, 'Are you sure you don't want to get on one of those nice ponies?' and every time came that same polite little sing-song reply from you, 'No, thank you'. Sometimes in life, Freddie, you can't win them all and you've got to take it on the chin when you get beaten by a more determined opponent!

* * *

I referred to your sleeping in the last chapter and how good it was after we got the 'baby whisperer' to sort out your routine. From when you were three months to just before you were two we were the smug parents with the 'incredible sleeping baby'. We couldn't join in those conversations with our friends who were having terrible broken nights with babies and toddlers who just refused to sleep through. We'd look at each other knowingly across the dinner table at these times, eyes smiling, a silent message passing between us ... 'Aren't we lucky to have the incredible sleeping baby?' Your dad loves his sleep and I was going through cancer treatment from when you were fourteen months old, so to be able to pop you in your cot, walk straight out and know you'd soon be off to enjoy a peaceful and full night of slumber was a great feeling.

But then of course you became more active and started to walk. You could stand up in your cot now and the base was dropped to the lowest level possible. Then, disaster of disasters, you worked out that if you stamped around in your baby sleeping bag long enough the poppers would come undone at the shoulders and your legs would be free for you to kick one up over the side of the cot and climb out. So we bought you a sleeping bag with a zip! But soon after, with those long legs of yours, not even a bag could stop you and like a little baby Houdini you'd be up and over those bars. The sleeping bag then became an issue when landing and a couple of times you reached the floor with a bump. There followed several mornings where you woke and cried at five, then I spotted you on the baby monitor halfway over the cot-prison bars and had to shout Daddy awake with 'QUICK! QUICK! HE'S GOING TO FALL'. He'd leap out of bed, looking super-confused after being woken from such a deep sleep, to rush into your room to catch you before you hit the (really quite cushioned with carpet) deck. There was nothing else for it. For safety reasons we were going to have to move you into your cot bed, AKA The Worst Decision We Ever Made. I think one of the best pieces of advice I can give you in this book, Freddie, if and when you decide to have children, is NEVER MOVE THEM OUT OF THEIR COTS! Do everything you can to keep them in there. Some of your little friends are still in their cots, a year after we had to move you into a bed, and I am so jealous.

It all started off well enough, and it was even kind of an exciting moment. Daddy got down the different bits we needed from the loft to switch your cot into a bed. We went shopping for your super-cute little duvet, pillow and new covers and approached the first night with a huge air of excitement. We'd put some cushions along the floor on the side of the bed in case you rolled out, and you looked so adorable when you got all snuggled up under your little duvet and went off to sleep. You barely moved all night. And the same the second night. We high-fived a successful transition from cot to bed. That was easy, we thought. Then I did something a little bit stupid.

You had always taken your naps in your pushchair. For some reason, even though you slept like the proverbial baby in your room at night, you just wouldn't settle in the day. But a cot bed was different, right? Wrong. There followed a frustrating hour or so where I'd put you in the bed and you'd climb straight out and follow me to the door. And we'd keep repeating this rather irritating little loop. But I've told you, I can be stubborn and I kept on trying. So what I was basically doing was showing you that you could get out of that little bed any time you wanted. And that's exactly what you started to do that night. We'd put a baby gate on your door to stop you wandering around in the night and falling down the stairs, and every time we'd try and leave the room you'd appear there the moment it shut. We'd try and do what the baby whisperer had advised and quietly take you back to bed, kiss you goodnight and leave the room again. But there's only so many times you can do that without losing the will to live. I was mid-radiotherapy at that point and really tired. And so we did all the wrong things because sometimes that is easier! This has escalated into us having to sit with you while you go to sleep, which can often take up to an hour as your busy little mind and body take a loooonnnng time to wind down. Then there was a period where you would wake throughout the night and cry or have night terrors, so one of us (Daddy) would have to come in to you, and at that time of night all he wanted to do was go back to sleep, so he'd end up on a mattress on the floor in there.

There were many suggestions from people to just let you 'cry it out'. It'll only take a few days, they said. It'll be worth it in the long run. But neither Daddy or I had the heart to let you cry for more than a few seconds. We want our boy to be happy and leaving you to cry alone in your room just seemed totally wrong. We knew we'd really thrown in the towel in this whole bedtime battle when we started using the big day bed in there, made up as a king-size bed, with your little duvet on one side and pillows and duvet on the other for when Daddy would invariably end up in your room at 3 a.m.! I hesitate to say it out loud, but I do think you've started to turn a corner recently. You still often take an hour to go off while one of us lies there listening to you chatter on about your day and when you try to delay sleeping by asking for apples, drinks, books and torches. But then you manage to sleep through the night with no further wake-ups and there have been an increasing number of mornings recently where I have woken with Daddy next to me in our bed! (He was in it so little for a while that you started calling it 'Mummy's bed'.)

Early on in the 'sleep routine' process we were encouraged to get you attached to some sort of 'comforter' that smelt of Mummy and would soothe you wherever you took it. Auntie Claire had given us a lovely grey-and-white elephant comforter when you came along, so we decided to use that and 'Mr Snuggles' was born. You soon became very attached to him, though you only ever want him when you're tired and need to go to sleep. You send yourself into a bit of a pre-sleep trance by rubbing his soft velvety material between your fingers and this is always the moment I know you're about to drop off. To avoid any of those awful 'We've lost Mr Snuggles' moments we bought about five of them. But somewhere along the line you have colonized all of them and generally insist on taking at least three of them to bed with you. Another delaying sleep tactic probably – 'I want other snuggles!' – but there is only one that you really like and I've no way of fathoming which it is. You know them by touch and I'm now too scared to wash them in case I do the wrong thing with your favourite!

You also love to have your arms tickled as you go to sleep, which is something both Mummy and Daddy used to love as children too. Now that your speech is so good you'll ask me, 'Will you tickle my arms, Mummy?' and if I try to stop you'll grab my hand and put it back on your palm for more tickles. These are the times I love most at the moment, where we are snuggled up on the giant bed with you about to go off to sleep and I can comfort you. I keep telling you how very much I love you in the hope you might retain some memories of this as you grow up. You keep telling me how much you miss me, like you know what's coming. But of course you can't know. It's just a lovely little thing you do at the moment. So when you can, try and delve back into your memories, Freddie, and picture Mummy laying face-to-face with you on the bed, tickling your arms and telling you how very, very much I love you. Always have and always will.

* * *

Aside from walking, the other big thing every parent looks forward to in a baby's first year is their first words. You were on the slower end of the scale for this, too busy running, jumping and climbing things for chit-chat. But I had my own personal speech therapist on hand in the guise of Auntie Claire and she said nothing worried her at all about your speech and communication. But it was something that concerned me for a time. I laugh about it now because over the last few months, as you approach your third birthday, we cannot get you to shut up! Formerly peaceful car journeys are now spent listening to you ask a million questions. You constantly parrot back everything we say so we have to be very careful with our language. And you are fast turning into a little chatterbox.

You went through what was a very cute stage of only saying one syllable of a word. But it wasn't always necessarily the first sound. Daddy became 'Dah' and Mummy became 'Mee'! I actually really like being called Mee as it made me feel different to all the other mums, mummies and mamas. My boy loved me so much he had created his own special name for me. Though I think when we were out and about people just thought you were some sort of baby-narcissist as you ran around shouting for 'Mee'!

You soon moved on to multi-syllable words though and I graduated from Mee to Mummy. Then you started forming longer and longer sentences and finishing your words with a flourish. You say so many things now that catch us by surprise at their complexity and level of understanding. Your dad and I often glance across at each other, eyebrows raised, wondering 'Where on earth has he learnt that?!' I think you do pick up a lot from the children's TV programmes you watch. We've probably given you more screen time than we should but obviously there's been a lot going on. We always thought before we had you that we wouldn't be those parents who stuck a phone in front of their children while they were out or let them watch TV shows. Idiots! It's often the only way to get a bit of peace and quiet, and like I say, you seem to learn a lot from these programmes.

Then there are the funny little turns of phrases you come out with, which leave us guessing where you've picked them up from. They're often the things we don't notice ourselves saying. But suddenly realize we do. We can easily spot the ones from Gran – 'shoo Bodie' – or your cousin Imogen – 'Come on, little one'. But some of the others are just a mystery. Many of your baby words we have kept on as our new Bland family vocabulary. For example, an orange will forever more be an 'uh-zhure', lawnmowers will stay as 'law-laws', cheese sandwiches to me and your daddy are now 'chee-fahs', fish fingers are 'fat-fees' and sausages are 'sos-jidges'. Arguably the most entertaining toddler misspeak happened on a walk out with Bodie when you insisted on calling a big stick a 'big dick'. Cue me and your dad doubled over, holding onto a tree for support with tears of laughter streaming down our faces. Maybe we won't keep that one in the Bland family language.

* * *

In the last chapter I told you how everyone thought you were the world's smiliest baby as you were always grinning away in your photos. It was so easy to get you to pose for the camera. Like all new parents, we've always be keen to document every moment. I even took a photo on the first of every month of your first year with you lying next to your teddy bear made out of Grandad Hodges' clothes for scale. In every picture (apart from the first couple before you'd developed the ability) you are grinning like the proverbial Cheshire Cat. Then bam, literally the moment you turned one, you developed an attitude and hated having your photo taken from then on. So now our cameras are full of photos of Daddy and I grinning away over-enthusiastically or pulling faces to try and make you smile while you sit between us with an enormous frown on your face! It's almost impossible to get a good family photo these days and if we do manage to get one of us all with eyes open, looking towards the camera and with a vague air of happiness about us, we cherish it.

* * *

After getting the bad news in April 2018 that my cancer was back, the summer that followed seemed like it had been sent to lift our spirits until a few weeks ago. It has been wall-to-wall sunshine with so little rain in the usually drenched North West that a hosepipe ban was threatened, something I'd not heard of since I was a child and certainly could never have expected would be possible around Manchester. For weeks and weeks it's felt like we've spent most of our time out in the garden together and I have loved it. You are so happy when you're running around outside and I always think the fresh air goes some way to tiring you out.

We are nearly there with my perfect garden set-up with our lovely corner sofa out on the decking underneath a large umbrella that's right next to that climbing frame we got you for your first birthday. I know I've hit middle age now, as when it's hot and sunny I'd much rather be in the shade than baking in the sun. My ideas of lazing on the sofa with a book or doing some writing are scuppered when you decide you want me to play with you. You are often to be found with your toolbox and hammer at the top of the slide fixing things. I am blaming Grumpy and his garage full of magic tricks for your obsession with fixing! Every time I get myself comfortable you shout over in your best 'Bob the Builder' foreman's voice, 'Come on, Mummy. Let's get busy!' and I get dragged off my lovely comfy sofa to help you.

It felt like the paddling pool was constantly out through the whole of June and July. Daddy had to keep emptying it every week or so and moving it around the lawn so as not to totally kill off the grass, although the heatwave was doing a good job of that on its own. I went a step up in our paddling-pool purchase this year – a large square one with seats in each corner! It was of course all for your benefit ... I will never admit that I spent more time in there reclining with a good book and cooling down than you ever did splashing around! I could just as easily supervise your play from the nice, cool paddling pool under the shade of the gazebo as anywhere else. I basically just let you dig up most of the borders with your garden tools and bury whatever you wanted (which reminds me to ask your dad to dig up the 'Toot-Toot' race-car you've just covered in earth out there). I have always had an affectionate nickname for you as you whirl around throwing toys about you in a frenzy of playtime ... my Feral Fred. Always happiest when making a mess and doing what you probably shouldn't!

This was the summer you also learnt the art of coercion to get what you want. You were very keen on a Magnum Mini – 'ice cream on a stick' as you referred to it. You'd ask for one by telling me how hot you were: 'I need a ice cream to cool down, Mummy.' What mother could say no to that logic? It meant I ended up eating a lot of ice cream too, because yes, it was hot, and you were right, ice creams do cool you down.

In May we had a lovely little mini 'holiday' to the Chatsworth International Horse Trials in Derbyshire. We usually pop over to the event for a day to watch the cross-country every year, but this summer you'd been chatting a lot about going on a holiday. We'd just bought you a sweet little Trunki ride-on case and we needed somewhere to use it. Seeing as you didn't know the difference between Chatsworth and the Caribbean, we decided on a visit to the horse trials, a night in a hotel near the estate, then a day on the Peak Rail steam train, as you are fully obsessed with trains and had never been on one.

This year you really enjoyed Chatsworth. It's a big three-day-event experience so you can watch all the disciplines starting with dressage, which features set moves for the horse and rider which have to be controlled and precise. Then comes the cross-country and the most fun bit to watch, as the riders put full trust in their horses' bravery to leap the enormous fixed fences around the course that snakes through the beautiful Chatsworth Estate. Then you can go down to the central showjumping ring and sit in one of the makeshift stands or just grab a spot around the fence and watch horse and rider work in concentration together to leap over huge wooden jumps that will fall at the merest tickle of a hoof. I say you enjoyed all this … you did love seeing the 'horseys', shouting 'STOP!' and 'Catch that horsey' as they galloped by on the cross-country course. But you kind of preferred eating ice creams and collecting sticks with Daddy! At least this gave Mummy some nice peaceful spectating time.

But your absolute favourite thing there was the bouncy castle. We hadn't tried you on one before and Daddy was convinced you wouldn't like it. There was a complicated queuing system where you had to stand in line with your money ready to pay and you weren't a fan of standing away from Mummy and Daddy. Then it was a little high for you to get up, so Daddy stepped over the fence that was meant to be keeping the adults out and gave you a leg up. We watched anxiously, wondering if you'd want to get straight off, but no, hallelujah! Once you worked out how to bounce you LOVED it. I had to watch through my hands a few times as you got a bit close to the older children, but you just watched what they were doing and copied it. When the whistle went to say your six minutes were up, all the other kids dutifully climbed down and went back to put their shoes on, but you just carried on bouncing away at the back. You looked so happy that your dad and I just chucked some more money at the man in charge and you carried on bouncing. We couldn't let you stay on there all day though as it would have bankrupted us, so the next time the whistle went the poor bouncy-castle man had to spend a good couple of minutes chasing you around it to hand you back to us. Now I look out for bouncy castles whenever we go to an event as I know they'll be a hit with my little Tigger.

A fun day had by all, we packed up and went to the hotel I'd let Daddy book. Normally I'm a bit of a control freak about holiday or hotel bookings as I like a certain standard and your dad doesn't always quite understand what that is! But the one he'd shown me looked good online. The main hotel was nice enough but we were told family rooms were in an annexe. No fancy hotel stay ever happened in a seventies annexe. The room was damp, dark and the bathroom had avocado accents on the tiles. It was meant to be a treat after receiving the bad news that my cancer was back and this room did not feel like a treat. It was made worse by your dad mentioning that as we were checking in someone else had said they didn't want their room and were leaving straight away. And this wasn't a cheap room. It was expensive and even I begrudge paying money for something that isn't worth it. After a quick ring around hotels near by, one called the Cavendish said they could accommodate us, so we checked straight out and headed there instead. Sometimes in life, Freddie, when you don't like something, you've got to change it. We could have stayed in that musty room complaining all night, but much better to take a decision to move on. Your dad walked out saying he felt empowered!

We headed to the Cavendish Hotel in Baslow and it couldn't have been more perfect if I had summoned it up in my imagination. It is on the Chatsworth Estate so the views overlooked the horse stabling in the fields and we could see all the owners' lorries parked up in the distance. The building itself is a light sandstone, the same colour as the main Chatsworth House. Inside, it is the perfect mix of country shabby chic. Luxurious enough to make it special but not so OTT as to make you feel out of place. The staff all wore tweed uniforms, which I loved, and they were so lovely to you. All the waiters smiled and played with you as you ran around with your helicopters. Our room was stunning and after a lovely dinner we settled you down to bed in your little bunk before having a glass of wine and gazing at the views of the croquet lawn out of the window. The next morning at breakfast there was high excitement as a helicopter came in to land on the helipad outside. Dad grabbed you and the two toy helicopters you already happened to have with you, and you were so excited to see the real-life version right in front of you.

I was so charmed with the hotel and its surroundings that I begged Daddy to stay another night there as we were having such a lovely time. He eventually relented, of course, even though it was a work night and would mean an early start in the morning. We had another amazing day taking you on the Peak Rail steam train which you loved, then heading back to the horse trials to watch some more of the cross-country. We went back to the hotel, where we'd had to move rooms as our original one was booked. We ended up with a huge four-poster bed that was so high there was a set of steps to climb up to it! There followed a slightly anxious night after you appeared at the top of the steps at some point in the early hours and jumped in with us. I had visions of you rolling out and falling four feet to the floor. But we survived the night intact. The next day I called the hotel to book our room for next year. It was something to aim for at the time, but it's unlikely I'll make it that far now. But I hope you and Daddy will go back there together and remember that wonderful happy family weekend we spent watching horses and riding trains. My spirit will always be with you, Freddie, in the places I love.

Chapter 10

GROWING UP WELSH

'm not sure whether any of my earliest memories of growing up in Wales are prompted by the old school photographs at Grandma's or whether they are real. This is one of the main things that worries me about leaving you so young; it's that you'll have no real memories of me and that is why I'm writing my life and soul down here for you, Freddie. My earliest memories that I know are real – because there are no photographs of the moment – were at Mama and Bampy's house (Grandma's parents) in a place called Pentre in the Rhondda Valley. It was a small terraced house on a long street of identical stone buildings. I would have been about your age because they both died not long after my third birthday and that gives me some little hope that you will retain some memories of me. I can remember eating soup at their dining table at the front of the house, searching for Opal Fruits sweets (now confusingly called Starburst) in their kitchen cupboards. And the time a robin flew into the house and got stuck behind the TV – most of the flapping that went on was done by Grandma and Mama!

I grew up in a little village called Creigiau which is about seven miles to the north-west of the capital city of Wales – Cardiff. The village was next to a quarry, which I think is the origin of its name as Craig in Welsh means 'rocks'. It was a fairly unremarkable village but a lovely, quiet place to grow up in. There was one petrol station and shop, and a Post Office that sold penny sweets – imagine that, sweets for a penny? They were the good old days. There was one pub in the centre of the village, The Creigiau Inn – a surprisingly uncreative name for a nation that can put words together without using vowels.

Grandma and Grandad Hodges bought our seventies four-bed – which back then would practically have been a newbuild – when I was just eight months old and they never left. They were very happy in their home at the bottom of a cul-de-sac and saw no reason to move on. It was a corner plot which had a fairly large garden. And even after Grandad Hodges died, and the house probably became a bit too much for Grandma to keep up, she always refused to leave because it was where all her happy memories had been made.

Whenever you look back at the summers of your youth, Fred, I hope they are the ones of eternal sunshine and happy playtimes that I remember. It's a good metaphor for life, I think, to remember more of the sunny times and forget about the miserable rainy days. I know it will perhaps be more difficult for you than for many of your peers, but I know there are so many of those sun- and fun-filled days ahead of you. And the times when you miss having Mummy there to hold you and to comfort you, remember you will always have a mummy who loves you more than anything in this world. That's a lot of love that I'm leaving behind with you, my darling, and I hope you always feel it around you.

Most of my summers were spent playing out by the roundabout outside our house with Uncle Matthew and the other children in the street. Summer holidays were usually taken in Devon, Cornwall or on the Isle of Wight in the caravan that Grandma and Grandad bought when I was five. Yes, we were those caravanners that drive other people mad on the motorway. As a child, I found the caravan quite exciting – like a little house on wheels. It had all the mod cons – a sofa and table, a gas hob, sink and even a fridge and TV! A real home away from home. Grandma would pack the cupboards full of wonderfully unhealthy eighties snacks like Monster Munch crisps and Club chocolate bars. And your Uncle Matthew and I would fight over who got to be on the top bunk of the sofa at the back that converted into beds. That was, of course, until we both grew quite a lot and realized the bottom bunk had way more room, then we'd squabble over who took ownership of that!

While my friends at school would be off on exotic holidays in Europe or further afield I would be living it up in the lap of caravan luxury anywhere from St Davids to Land's End. You see Grandma was always terrified of flying and point-blank refused to get on a plane. Also, we always had a dog (I think Grandma used them as a handy excuse!) and this was in the days before dog walkers and pet sitters and she just couldn't bear the thought of putting them in kennels. So we were always packed up in Grandad Hodges' old Sierra with the dog in the boot, the caravan on the back and a hankering in my heart to go somewhere more exotic. And I haven't even mentioned the time the dog vomited over the back seat and all over my new Sindy horse. I think that's why I used to get in as many trips abroad as possible as I got older, to make up for the lack of travelling in my youth. I hope I don't sound ungrateful though, Freddie, because I had some wonderful times on those trips in the caravan going on rides in theme parks, hanging out at the beach, drinking Orangina on the jetties and attempting some fishing and crabbing with Grandad. The only occasion we actually caught anything was the one time we went out fishing on a proper little boat a bit further out to sea. Grandad Hodges was thrilled with his haul of four mackerel, letting out one of his customary foghorn impressions (we will come on to Grandad's sound repertoire later!) before we came back into port. I was fascinated by these fish and watched closely as Grandad gutted them, really very professionally for a man who spent most of his time looking at an empty hook. But I became a little green around the gills myself after seeing one of their last meals emerge and point-blank refused to eat any of our catch, so I was stuck with beans on toast for dinner.

The other big event from the summers of my youth was the Creigiau Carnival organized by the members of the Creigiau 23 men's dinner club (yes, Fred, there was a time when dinner clubs were men-only events – shocking!), of which Grandad was a member. He would seem to spend a lot of time helping with the beer tent. Much like the Knutsford May Day there would be a float procession around the village with a different theme each year, headed up by a carnival queen and her attendants. The route would process down to the recreation ground which would be full of lucky-dip stalls, with a bit of welly-wanging and 'splat the rat' thrown in for good measure. Every year Grandma would put me in some really rather good fancy dress. There was the time I went as a tube of Smarties, the year she covered me in strips of pink crêpe paper in a brilliant resemblance of Mr Messy and the occasion when Grandad and his balsa wood got involved and they made me a full-blown ladybird shell to carry on my back. I'm pretty sure I won the fancy-dress competition that year – and if I didn't, then I definitely should have done!

As sunny as the summers would be, in my fuzzy memories of old, winters were always cold and snowy and revolved mainly around Christmas. The spindly pine tree I talked about earlier would go up in the lounge, with decorations that Grandma still uses now. Then Uncle Matthew and I would fight over where was the best place to ask Father Christmas to leave us our presents. I favoured between the TV and the footstool.

I was obsessed with My Little Ponies, which probably explains why I loved horses so much as I grew up, and anything from the Sindy and Barbie range of dolls. The glitzier and more gaudy the ballgown the better! I really had very unrefined tastes in clothing back in those days. Crystal Barbie and Peaches 'n Cream Barbie had enough synthetic sheeny fabric and ruffles to make even the most ardent eighties fan turn away in horror. But I loved them, that is until I was a few years older and into that phase of 'Let's give Barbie a buzz cut' – we all go through it.

If it wasn't me breaking my toys and treasured possessions, then it was your Uncle Matthew. He's a bit of an engineer, so he decided to take apart my lovely red ghetto blaster (an eighties thing, look it up, along with cassette tapes!) to see how it worked. It never got put back together. He borrowed my prized lilac Bianca bike. It came back with a buckled front wheel. Then there was the time that he and our cousin, Uncle Robbie, thought it was hilarious to keep throwing my teddy bears out of my upstairs bedroom window, and as I sprinted up and down the stairs rescuing each one another would go for the skydive just as I stepped into the bedroom! And let's not mention the time Uncle Matthew and his friend got bored of playing darts on his new dartboard and decided to start chucking them in my direction as I cowered behind a bed. But for all his torturing me as I child, there were times I appreciated his company and we played companionably on his road playmat, each pretending our car could jump like those in *The Dukes of Hazzard* – our favourite Saturday-night viewing at the time.

For Freddie

I had always so wanted you to have siblings, Freddie. We'd just starting trying for a brother or sister for you when I was diagnosed with cancer and even then I didn't give up hope. Cancer treatments can wreak havoc with your fertility, so I insisted on having a round of IVF before I started chemo. You do have four little embryonic brothers and sisters in a freezer somewhere in Manchester. I would have loved to have had three children altogether, as I always think there is safety in numbers. And I'm so sorry, Fred, that I wasn't able to give you a sibling. It breaks my heart sometimes when I see you trying to play with other children at the park. You so want to get involved in their games, but haven't quite developed the right chat yet. Shouting 'NEH-NAH NEH-NAH' in their faces is usually your opening gambit. I'm sure your banter will improve with time. And we will always stay the three best friends; we don't need anyone else to make us complete. You were always more than enough for me. I'm so glad you have your three cousins living just around the corner and that little Barney will always be in the same school year as you. I can picture you now, riding your bike around there to play. I hope they will fill the gap left behind by those babies we dreamed of having but that never sparked into life in the way that you, my beautiful Fred, did.

* * *

The primary school that I went to in Creigiau was bilingual, with a Welsh section and an English section that were each taught in their own language. We all came together for assemblies in the main hall, where we'd sing songs in both languages as Mrs Morse banged away perhaps a little TOO enthusiastically on the piano. But beyond this daily meeting the two sides of the school had very little to do with each other, apart from the odd little taunt of calling the Welsh section children 'Welsh cakes' which would be rebutted with the equally cheeky 'English cakes'!

I always found it odd that we were never officially taught the Welsh language until we started comprehensive school. Way too late for me to start learning such a complicated language. And that is why I have excellent Welsh pronunciation but can't string a sentence together. I hope that Grandma will help to teach you the proper way to sound a double 'L' in Welsh, by putting your tongue to the top of your mouth. And that you won't forever call our wedding venue 'Lan-goyd' Hall like your dad does!

This is a good time to mention 'Welsh-isms', Fred, as you may not learn them anywhere else. These are classic Welsh idioms that generally say the same thing in more than one way. For example:

'I'll be there now in a minute.'
'Whose coat is that jacket?'
'Whose boots are those shoes?'
'I went to get my bike and there it was! Gone!'

For a country supposedly filled with beautiful singers we can really murder the English language.

* * *

As I've mentioned, I was always a very shy child growing up. I'm not sure why but I was never very confident. But shyness is often mistaken for being aloof and I think many kids in school just thought I was a bit stand-offish. This is probably where I began to get that misguided notion that anyone I didn't know well didn't like me very much. People who didn't know me very well would think I was quiet and didn't talk, while my best friends couldn't shut me up!

On all personality tests I've done since I score very highly on introversion and empathy. I always prefer being in a smaller group and can find big social events quite tiring as they take a lot of effort on my part to 'switch it on' and be chatty. I've got much better at it as the years have gone on, so much so people are shocked now when I tell them I'm shy. An introverted broadcaster is a fairly rare beast; most are normally right up the extrovert scale. But you know me, Freddie, I like to break the mould and do the opposite of what people think! I can see already you are way more confident than Mummy. Despite little episodes of shyness when you were a baby and not liking loads of people in your face at once – I mean who does like that?! – now you will go and try and chat to anyone we come across, adults and children, usually to proudly waggle your new toy in their face. The one thing I always said I wanted for you when you were born was for you to be confident, as it's the personality trait that has most eluded me in my life. And I know that Daddy and all the love of our families around will help you grow into a confident and happy little boy. Children, I am told, are very resilient. Despite living through such a tragic event as losing your mum when you are so young, you can still go on to do wonderful and amazing things. And I so wish that after this horrible start, you enjoy a charmed existence forever more.

Being shy and quiet meant I was often quite softly spoken and I would drive your grandad mad by almost muttering things under my breath so he couldn't hear what I was saying! Then there was the time I nearly missed out on winning a massive jar of sweets in a skittles competition on a caravan holiday one year. As they announced the winner, 'Rachael Rogers?', and nobody came forward it turned out it was actually me who had won, but with me giving my name so quietly they had missed that I'd said 'Hodges'! Obviously this softly spoken period got fixed as I did more and more newsreading and voice training, and learnt to speak more clearly, enunciate my words properly and project my voice more.

This was also the time I began to lose my Welsh accent. It was never a strong one to start with and I often call myself an 'accent chameleon' as I will pick up ways of speaking from those around me. Hang out with a bunch of English girls at uni – I'd sound English. Send me to Australia for a few months and suddenly I'd be greeting you with a 'g'day'. I'm sure if I looked it up it would have something to do with my empathetic side and wanting to fit in with others. I kind of miss having a Welsh accent as it's part of my heritage. One time on St David's Day (1 March – wear your leek and daffodil with pride on that day, Freddie!) I wore a red dress with a daffodil pin on my chest to read the sports news on the BBC News Channel. A major network news presenter and correspondent, who shall remain nameless but has a reputation for teasing, called me a 'plastic Welshy' because I didn't sound Welsh. How very dare he! I argued that I hadn't lived there for many years, so he pointed out neither had the legendary news presenter Huw Edwards and he still had his Welsh lilt. Yep, fair enough, he won that one! I hope you don't ever feel the need to fit in like I did, Fred. I would love you to have the confidence to not even take these sort of things into consideration.

Now at school in Wales we would go up a level from your basic daffodil on St David's Day and go to class dressed in full Welsh costume. For the girls this involved a slightly bizarre-looking flat-topped black hat with white lace hanging from the brim, plus an itchy woollen shawl pinned around our shoulders over a pinafore dress with white apron. The overall look was less high fashion and more high farce. Want to make farcical look even funnier? Dress your dog in this way! I once told a radio colleague I'd done this just as pictures flashed up on the

TV outside our studio of kids wearing national dress on St David's Day. I have never had someone look at me so incredulously as Paulina did that day and it was the trigger for my second most hysterical time on the radio after the 'Randy Bumgardener' incident. I was meant to be reading the news and Paulina the sport, and because of the way the local station was set up then we had to pre-record one bulletin before doing another one live. Well, after the 'dog in the Welsh costume' revelation we couldn't even sit in the same studio without crying with laughter. It got so time-critical that Paulina had to wait outside the studio while I read my news before I dashed out and she sat down to read the sport without our eyes meeting and setting us off again. For at least a week afterwards we couldn't look directly at each other without bursting into uncontrollable laughter.

* * *

I was always fairly musical as a child and had piano lessons from the age of about seven after Grandma and Grandad Hodges shelled out what was a fairly large amount of money at the time on a beautiful polished-mahogany upright piano. Every week I'd have to leave my friends playing in the park in the centre of Creigiau and head over to Mrs Gribble's house which overlooked it. She was a lovely lady and a very talented musician who played for the Welsh National Orchestra. Her house was beautifully furnished and I did all my lessons on the mini-grand piano in her front room with her Siamese cats sat around us eyeing me suspiciously and, I felt, judging my piano-playing skills. She always bought me beautiful music-themed presents for Christmas and the end of term – a treble-clef brooch or a notebook decorated with musical notes. I worked my way up through the grades until I reached the heady heights of Grade 5 and gave it all up.

I would love to say I'm a talented musician, Fred, but it would not be true, though I am a step or two up from your tone-deaf Grandad Hodges! I always say I would like to be able to sing. I can hold a tune but that's about as good as it gets. So it's nice to still be able to play the piano and read music. Whenever I'm at Grandma's house I get out all my old music books and if I don't think about it too closely, and just let my hands glide over the keys, I can still play them just as well as I did back in Mrs Gribble's house. Being able to play an instrument and read music can give you great pleasure, Freddie, and I'd love it if you were to learn how to play and read music in whatever form that may take. I've told Daddy he needs to pay for lessons if you want them!

As I grew from little girl into teenager, my confidence was also knocked by a rather bad run of hairstyles from the ages of ten to thirteen. I'd always wanted long hair, in fact I've just had super-long and beautiful hair extensions put in, as princess hair was on my 'bucket list'. By the time I was ten it had grown to just over shoulder length and had been bleached by the summer sun into a pleasing sandy colour. Then Grandma stepped in and I remember so clearly her saying 'It looks like rats' tails, you need a cut', before marching me off to the old ladies' hairdresser up the road. Well, I'm not sure what kind of cut they were going for but I ended up with what can only be described as a short, uneven moptop. All my beautiful blonde ends were snipped away, each chunk floating down to the hairdresser's floor taking a little bit of my broken heart with it. I hated that lop-sided crop. I think it is too generous to describe it as a 'hairstyle'. Grandma told me it looked great, as mothers always do. But the real test came when I walked down the road to meet my friend Rebecca, who was a lovely person and wouldn't have said anything horrible on purpose. She'd been looking at me blankly as I strolled down to meet her. Then as I got closer her eyes lit up in recognition as she exclaimed, 'Oh, it's you! I thought it was a boy coming down the road.' Excellent. Not the look every ten-year-old who really wants princess hair is going for. I think that cut is the reason I've kept my hair long for my whole adult life.

The other hairstyle that scarred me for life, and I cringe when looking back on pictures of it, was the year of 'the perm'! In the late eighties it was quite the fashion to get a permanent wave put in your hair with the use of curlers and chemicals that smelt of rotten eggs. A couple of girls at school had had them and so I begged Grandma to let me have one too. She eventually relented and off to the hairdresser we went. There were different types of perm and the one I really wanted was called a spiral perm, but I didn't know how to describe it to the hairdresser at the time. She cut my hair first, just as another lady walked in with the exact type of curl I wanted. I pointed her out to the hairdresser only to be told that woman had hair all the same length and the hairdresser had just finished putting layers into mine. Ah. What I was then left with was a kind of bushy, fuzzy, wavy mullet. I had no idea about using any products to tame it, so it mostly just looked fluffy! In my first year of comprehensive school photos that mullet is front and centre, you really couldn't miss it. Perhaps this is why I'm so fussy about your hair, Freddie, and perhaps you won't thank me for keeping it too long in the future. But for now, your gorgeous little moptop stays, nice and long!

* * *

I would describe myself as a little easily led through my teenage years – always impressed by people with big, bold personalities. I wish, looking back, that I had more confidence in myself back then and the courage of my convictions. I really hope that you will have that, Freddie, that you will know yourself and be bold enough to follow your own path and not get stuck in the crowd. It is much better to be focusing on your own way forward in life than worrying about what other people think about it, like I did. You've only got yourself and those you love to please. What anyone else thinks is irrelevant. It's often easier said than done, but this is advice I wish I'd had through my school years. The only boss of you is you, my Fred.

There is very little to do in a small village in South Wales, so my friends and I started branching out into Cardiff and nightclubbing at way too young an age. This was back in the day, when it was pretty easy to fake an ID, and that was if you even needed it as we could all dress up and look older than our years. Never be in too much of a rush to grow up, Freddie. There is plenty of time in your twenties for going out and having fun. I wish I had waited until I was older to experience these things, but I was always in a hurry through life in my teens, rushing on to the next stage before I was really ready to get there. I would much rather you followed in your dad's footsteps and had fun with your friends making up dance routines to 5ive tunes than spending time in bars. You are only young once and you have plenty of time ahead for being a grown up. And once you get there it is never as fun as you think. Being an adult involves quite a lot of responsibility and dull life admin.

Despite the odd weekend trip out to nightclubs in town, I was mostly very studious at school. A strange combination of both rebel and swot! I studied quite hard for my GCSEs – I had a colour-coded revision timetable and everything – and I ended up with nine grade A-Cs including my one A* in geography. Exams are important but only as a stepping stone to get onto the next rung of the educational ladder if that is the path you choose. No one has asked me in years what I got in my GCSEs or A levels or degree – it was a first, by the way. So work hard at your studies but remember it is not the be-all and end-all.

During my breaks between studious moments, me and a few friends had taken to leaving school 'early' on a Wednesday afternoon and skipping our art class. Uncle Matthew was driving and in college at this point, so he would swing by in my Grandma and Grandad's Astra and take us home to Creigiau. One week we arrived home to a flashing light on the answer-machine. This used to be a separate box next to the phone that would record messages. I decided to listen, and horror of horrors it was a message from my head of year, a fairly strict man called Mr Pearce, asking why I was not in school that afternoon and inviting them in for a chat with him! Well, I did what anyone else would do in this situation … panicked, cried and swiftly pressed delete on the message. I obviously wasn't that much of a rebel because I was terrified of what was going to happen. So I decided to keep Grandma out of the loop altogether and go on a charm offensive with Grandad. This started with me asking him if he wanted to go out riding on the horses that weekend. Halfway round, I told him about the message and pleaded with him not to tell Grandma. He sagely nodded and said, 'Ah, I wondered why you were so keen to come out riding'! He took the news of my bunking off school very well, agreed to go in to chat to Mr Pearce and that was the last time I ever cut classes at school.

* * *

It was while I was at comprehensive school that it began to dawn on me what a slow eater I was. I'd go into the canteen with friends and despite only having a hotdog – this was the late eighties, so that practically counted as health food – they'd always wolf down their lunches and be ready to leave while I was barely halfway through. I'd have to beg my friends to stay sitting with me as I hated to be left there eating on my own – it felt very exposed! I've already mentioned what a slow eater Grandad

Hodges was and I was very much his daughter. And you are the next in the generational line for slow eating. You can take hours over your dinner, distractedly shoving in the odd handful of peas here or twist of pasta there. You are basically an all-day grazer, keeping your food levels topped up. We have the same approach to food not touching – I think I should start using one of your toddler separator plates! I don't like it when the sauce gets on the salad or the salad dressing leaks into the rice. Your dad always laughs at me because I always have to leave something on the plate at the end of the meal and I'm not even sure why I do it. Or indeed what the offending piece of food has done.

* * *

When I was sixteen I went through one of the most traumatic events of my life that would have long-lasting effects on my mental health into adulthood. On a night out with friends I got into the back of an old-style Mini car to travel down from the neighbouring village of Pentyrch and back to Creigiau. This was a car that was designed to take four people, so it was overloaded with three of us in the back. This was also in the days before it was mandatory to wear seatbelts in the back of cars and there were none to keep us safe in this Mini. As we drove down the twisty road, everybody chatting loudly, the car suddenly veered to the right, across the wrong side of the road, and hit the hedge that ran alongside it. It was only later, as I analysed and reanalysed exactly what had happened – part of the coping process – that I worked out the car had then briefly skidded on its side, scraping the skin on the arm of the lad in front almost down to the bone. It then flipped onto its roof and spun violently, flinging out the three of us untethered in the back with centrifugal force.

I remember so clearly the feeling of flying through the air and landing with a sickening thud on the tarmac before skidding to a halt. I must have passed out briefly, as I came to and lifted my head from the road to see my arms splayed out at a very unnatural angle in front of me and panicked that they were badly broken. I gingerly tried to stand up and realized they still seemed to work. I lifted up one of my scraped and bloodied hands to touch my forehead and could feel a huge egg-shaped swelling in the centre, just below my hairline. I of course was not aware of the huge hole in the middle of it from which blood was pouring down onto my T-shirt. I stood in the dark in that unlit road and realized my friend was calling for me to help her get out from a hedge on the side of the road. I looked down at my feet to see I was now only wearing one shoe. How could I help her if I only had one shoe? I wondered in my concussed state, as I suddenly felt woozy and decided to sit down. Just before I passed out, I was aware of a car driving down the road, slowly picking its way through the debris of car parts and people and driving on without stopping. Never be that person, Freddie, always be the one who is prepared to stop and help those in need.

Next thing I knew I was being picked up and put into another car, that of some other friends who were travelling the same route as us but a few minutes behind. They were going to take us to their house just around the corner and call an ambulance, but I pleaded with them in my befuddled state to take us straight to the hospital up the road, as at this point I still thought I could get out of this without telling your grandparents! They kindly did as I asked and also stopped me from lighting a cigarette on the way as my clothes were soaked in petrol. So I laid my battered and bleeding head up against the car window, leaving a blood-splatter artwork that Jackson Pollock would have been proud of. We must have given the hospital staff quite a shock arriving unannounced in A&E bruised and bleeding, some of us quietly shaking in shock, others hyped up and wailing like banshees. I ended up with a huge L-shaped scar across the top of my head that, for the next few years, people would stare at and study as they spoke to me instead of looking me in the eye. The way it was stitched back together meant my hairline was never straight again, a minor thing that always really bothered me nonetheless. I had deep grazes to the skin on the back of my forearms and required further operations to pull chunks of the glass windscreen out of them. From head to foot there was no part of my body that was not grazed and scarred in some way.

The car crash profoundly shocked me, snatching away much of my innocence as a sixteen-year-old and giving me the early realization that bad things happen in this world that we don't have any control over. I suffered from post-traumatic stress disorder afterwards and for years couldn't go to sleep in a bed on my own or with the light off. Some nights I would even take my duvet into Grandma and Grandad's room and snuggle up on the floor in there. It was shortly after this that I began to experience panic attacks, which have been a lifelong struggle for me to control. I had some counselling afterwards but was always too shy to open up and really get the benefit from it. But as with my cancer treatment now, Freddie, at some point you have to dig deep and just carry on when these awful things happen. Just keep putting one foot in front of the other because that's the only option.

Around the time I finished my GCSEs I began going through my 'obstinate phase'. Let's call it being a teenager! Despite often worrying about what people think of me, I also do not like to be told what to do. A bit like you, Fred, though you seem to have started this phase alarmingly early. I'd decided I was too cool to return to school for sixth form and that I wanted to go to the college on the other side of town where your uncle had gone. The 'red rag to the bull' moment came when my lovely form teacher at Radyr Comprehensive boldly said, 'Oh Rachael, you'll definitely be back for sixth form year,' and I thought to myself, 'I definitely won't!' This is not a strategy I would advise you to follow, Freddie. It was another example of me cutting off my nose to spite my face, as I often wished in the couple of years following that I'd remained in the safe and cosy confines of Radyr sixth form with my friends Rachel, Tracy and Bethan, who'd all stayed on and were having a great time not wearing uniforms. And of course it meant I missed out on another teenage rite of passage, the sixth-form ball. This was way before the days when anyone tried to call them 'proms' and parents spent thousands on expensive dresses and tacky stretch limos for their precious children. No, this was more of a long black number from Dorothy Perkins and a string of your mum's pearls kind of affair. But it was held in the City Hall in the centre of Cardiff and I always regretted not being in that photo with all of my friends on the steps of the hall. It's never a good thing to think you're too cool for school, Fred!

So, off I trotted to Coleg Glan Hafren in Rumney to study A levels in English, geography and media studies – a subject that wasn't on offer at Radyr. I made a few friends but as I was still pretty shy at this stage I spent much of the time being overwhelmed by the size of the college I found around me. But it did me good to get out of my comfort zone and doing media studies alongside all the work experience I was taking on in radio and TV at the time confirmed to me that I definitely wanted to go into journalism. A course that let you study *Pretty Woman* seemed like a pretty good one to me! The two years passed by in a flash, another colour-coded revision timetable was taped up on a cork board at Grandma and Grandad's house, and I felt confident and prepared as I scribbled down my answers to the exam questions. Of course when the time rolled around to go and collect my results I had talked myself down to Cs, Ds and Es and convinced Grandma and Grandad of the same. So it came as a pleasant surprise when I came running out clutching my exam results slip proudly bearing the letters A, B, B, and with my place on my first-choice course to study Journalism, Film and Broadcasting at Cardiff University secured.

* * *

One of the silver linings of the awful car accident I had had was the compensation money that allowed me to buy my first car. While flash friends told me to buy convertible Escorts and the like, I decided to be sensible and buy a brand-new car that would last me as long as possible. So just after my eighteenth birthday I went down to James & Jenkins motors in Llandaff North to pick up my pride and joy. My little silver Vauxhall Corsa may not have been the coolest of cars but it was all mine and it was all shiny and unsullied by the bad driving of others. They'd even put a big red bow across the bonnet ready for me to collect it. Your uncle laughed at its skinny little tyres, likening them to four digestive biscuits! And he christened it 'The Roller Skate', a name that would stick with it for the next ten years of our driving partnership.

That car represented independence to me. I never had to ask your grandparents' permission to borrow the car. It gave me freedom to get around at university and when I went into full-time work it meant I was all set up with my wheels, skinny as they might have been, ready to go. It had a nippy little 1.4-litre engine which on a car of that size wasn't shabby. This was in the days before any mod cons, so there weren't any electric windows, air conditioning and the like. But I loved that car and we continued our wonderful driving association right up until the time I moved to London a good ten years later.

I was working at BBC London at the time which was then based on the beautiful Marylebone High Street. There were only a couple of staff parking spaces right out of the back of the studios. Vanessa Feltz was presenting the mid-morning show at the time and one day word got round the newsroom that poor Vanessa had nearly been overcome by a waft of petrol fumes that were being blown into her studio from somewhere outside. How awful, I thought, I'm glad I don't have to sit in that studio today. I dashed out when I'd finished my shift at 1 p.m. and jumped in the Roller Skate to drive back to Wales to see Grandma and Grandad Hodges. Just as I was about to turn the key in the ignition, I suddenly got a very strong waft of petrol and realized that it might have been the Skate trying to poison Vanessa with those fumes. I got out and nervously looked under the car to see a large pool of petrol underneath it on the floor. Ah. Bugger. I went back inside to call the breakdown people and there started an afternoon of the most frustrating nature.

It turned out that the fuel tank had cracked, and where fuel is involved nobody seems to want to pick up the car. The breakdown van came and said it would need a lorry as he couldn't tow it. A flatbed lorry arrived and turned away, again proclaiming he couldn't take it and I'd have to call the fire brigade. The fire brigade said their only responsibility was to wash down the area where the petrol was. After six hours of going around in circles I called the first breakdown man back and he took pity on me. He said he needed a car to do up for his son, so if I was happy for him to take it away then he would. I was so relieved I could have hugged him. So I stood on that little road out the back of the Marylebone High Street studios and waved goodbye to my faithful old Roller Skate, never the most glamorous or stylish of cars, but a workhorse that had seen me through much of my youth. I hope the breakdown man's son got as many happy times out of that Corsa as I did.

* * *

Before we leave my childhood years behind, Freddie, I guess I should tell you about my first proper trip abroad. I had been on bus trips with school to Normandy and Austria, but in the summer that I was seventeen I flew to Majorca on my first fully-fledged 'girls trip'. We stayed in a pretty little apartment complex centred around a large pool in Palma Nova, right next door to that Mecca of tacky holidays, Magaluf! I went with Auntie Jo and Rachel for two weeks of sunshine. Now the first big hurdle to overcome was getting on a plane for the first time. This just happened to be exactly a year to the day after my car accident, so nerves were a little fraught. But this was back in the day when you could smoke on planes. Can you imagine, Fred? With all the safety measures in place now, and knowing how unhealthy it was, they'd just pull a curtain – like that was going to keep the smoke away from the non-smoking section – and let everyone puff away in the back. I should plead with you at this point, Freddie, never to take up smoking. There are very few times in the book that I will express a firm opinion on what I want from your future, because it is all yours to learn and explore, but please never smoke. I started smoking to try and fit in with a gang down at the riding school and it was a habit I struggled to give up until I met your daddy. Such was the esteem I held him in before we'd even got together, I decided I had smoked my last cigarette on the last day of my ski holiday and never smoked again after we got together. It's an awful habit and I always question whether it contributed to me getting cancer at such a young age. You only get one body to see you through this life, Fred, so make sure you keep it as healthy as you can.

Magaluf is definitely not the kind of place one keeps a healthy body as I was about to find out. I'd never even had a second's thought about my weight growing up and going through comprehensive school. I'd always been slim, though not skinny, and with a flat stomach. I was active and into running, cross-country and swimming. Turns out none of that will help you when you exist for two weeks purely on cheap, brightly coloured alcohol of indeterminate origin, crisps and food you choose from a slightly grubby-looking laminated picture outside a 'restaurant', all of which seemed to involve a lot of chips and very few vegetables. I put on a stone in those two weeks that I struggled to shift for the rest of my adult life. Turns out fat is not included in the notorious old phrase 'What goes on tour stays on tour'! The lady who was staying in the apartment next door with her older children did nothing to slow the fattening of the prize calves. She had brought with her numerous packs of frozen bacon and the like, which to be fair, when you saw the reality of the food out and about, seemed like a damn good idea. She kept handing them over to us every few days while muttering under her breath about never letting her daughters go on holiday on their own at our age.

One of the other quick learning curves on that holiday was how much stronger the Majorcan sun was compared to the English one I'd been used to when wrapped up in a towel on a freezing, rainy beach in Cornwall somewhere. I barely even remember using sun cream in my youth. So when my friends had advised me to make sure I put the factor 20 on well (I didn't want to go too overboard – I needed to tan!), I thought I had … until I woke up the next morning feeling like I'd been dipping my feet into a pool of flames overnight. I hadn't even thought to rub it on the tops of my feet and spent the next week trying to cover the burnt bits in sunblock until the rest of my leg caught up on the colour match.

Despite all the bright lights, tackiness, dancing and cheap drinks of 'The Strip' in Magaluf being fun at times, my favourite parts of the holiday were sitting on the terrace of our apartment, looking out over the pretty swimming pool area with a glass of cheap Spanish wine putting the world to rights with Auntie Jo and Rach. And the right friends are the only component you need to make a good holiday. My best and oldest friends in life who I met growing up in Wales – Jo, Rach, Trace, Erica, Lucy and Laura – are still my best mates now. Though we all left Wales and settled in the far corners of the globe, when we're back together we pick up just where we left off. We had a night out in Cardiff recently to celebrate a) all being in the country at the same time and b) our thirty years of friendship, and it was just like we were gossiping back on the 'quad' in Radyr Comp. I love those girls and know they'd do anything for me and me for them. They've all been there for me throughout my illness to talk, vent, whatever. And given the opportunity I would have loved to have been around longer to do the same for them. But I know I can rely on them to look after you and Daddy when I have gone.

I hope you meet some wonderful friends as you grow up, Freddie, and always hold on tight to the good ones. You'll be able to spot them easily. They're the ones who will have your back in any given situation but won't expect anything in return. They're the ones who will give you 'honest' advice and not just say what you want to hear. They're the ones who won't make jokes at your expense (unless you do something really funny, like slide off a swing with your toddler son on your lap with a TV camera pointed directly at you for a shoot and end up like a beetle stranded on its back … which may or may not have happened this week). And they are the ones who'll be able to make you laugh until the tears are streaming down your face and your tummy muscles start to hurt.

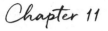

THE HODGES

I do so hope that you still have my mum, your grandma, around whenever you're reading this, Freddie. She adores you and you're always giving her the biggest cuddles whenever you see her. Or 'cwtches' as we call them in Wales – a word she gets you using every time she comes up to visit us from Cardiff!

Gran and Grumpy were always amazing with how much time they gave up to look after you when I went back to work part-time when you were eleven months old. It meant we didn't have to waste money we didn't really have on expensive nursery fees. And they get to keep very busy with you and your cousin Barney trying to wreck the joint, before his older sisters, Imogen and Matilda, get home from school to help!

So every few weeks Grandma will come up for a week or so at a time and take over some of the Freddie Day Care! She has always wanted to help as much as possible in your upbringing and care, though has to make the 182-mile drive up from Cardiff with Tilly, her golden retriever, to lend a hand. At any age the drive up the M5/M6 can be a daunting one, but when you're seventy-three and of a slightly nervous disposition then it can be terrifying. But Grandma has got it all down to a fine art now and while you'd never say her driving skills challenged those of Lewis Hamilton, you'd bet on them rivalling those of his gran! Whenever she arrives at the door, with an excited and barking Tilly leading the way, your eyes light up, you throw your arms around her and give her the 'heart-melter', 'Grandma, I missed you', and I know you have.

Grandma's real name is Gayna Hodges, née Evans. She was born and brought up in the Rhondda Valley in South Wales in a town called Pentre. The Rhondda was synonymous with coal mining back then and her grandfather Herbert Russ and his brothers had moved there from Somerset some time during the 1890s to work down the mines. Daddy always teases me that I'm not really Welsh, as Grandad Hodges was English (though actually more Welsh than most, but we'll get onto that) and Grandma's family are English one generation back. I of course tell him he's wrong! Interesting piece of family-tree trivia for you, Freddie: Herbert's brother was a Frederick and his first son – Grandma's uncle – was a Fred, born in 1893, so just a couple of your ancestors that your name was a nod to.

Grandma grew up on Volunteer Street in Pentre in one of the identical three-bedroom stone terrace houses that snaked their way up and down the rugged mountains of the valleys. She was the only child of Annis and Jack Evans, my Mama and Bampy. They were married for sixteen years before your grandma was born and had thought they couldn't have children. Then World War Two broke out. Bampy had flat feet and wasn't allowed to fight, so joined the building volunteers and worked in Plymouth for a lot of the war. They took in a young evacuee from London called Beryl, who lived with them until 1946, and perhaps that helped Mama to relax about having children because just as the war ended in 1945 – at what was back then, for a first-time mother, the grand old age of thirty-nine – she had Mum. My mum, your Grandma Gayna.

Mining work was still the predominant form of employement in the valleys and Grandma grew up used to seeing the blackened faces of the colliers as they made their way home for a bath – there was never anything so modern as a shower in the mines. There was a real close-knit community in the Rhondda and Grandma, despite being an only child, grew up with a huge family around her. In total, four of the houses in Volunteer Street were taken up by members of the Russ family, with more living the streets near by. Grandma was particularly close to her cousins, Auntie Theresa and Uncle Greg, who lived a few doors down with her mum, sister, Aunt Dillys. She always said that they were so close growing up they were like siblings not cousins. This is what I hope we have created here in Knutsford for you, Freddie, with Gran and Grumpy and Auntie Claire and Uncle Mark living just around the corner. I have lovely visions of you playing with all your cousins over there or at our house or riding your bikes in the streets between. And of you and Barney setting off for your first day at primary school together, two ready-made little buddies who will look out for each other for life.

* * *

Grandma eventually left the Rhondda to go and work for Post Office Telephones in Cardiff and that is where she met Grandad – David Hodges. Her desk was opposite his and she says he was fun and full of mischief – that's the Grandad I know! That was in 1962, and they started dating at the end of 1965 and got married in St Peter's Church in Pentre in 1967. They briefly moved between a few different houses before coming to land in our house in Creigiau and, as I told you earlier, deciding never to move from there again!

It took a little while for your Uncle Matthew and me to come along, but eventually we did in 1975 and 1978. After we had arrived, Grandma then devoted her life and time to being a mum. And she was a brilliant one. She would have a few outside interests like the choir, but Grandma said her family were her pastime and she didn't need anything else to occupy her. Hey, worrying about me and your Uncle Matthew was a full-time job! I've already told you that Grandma is a full-time worrier – she dedicates herself to this with some passion. It meant that throughout my teenage years she would always offer to drop me and my friends off or pick us up from nights out at any time. I would quite often call these lifts in, as taxis were expensive! So Grandma would be roused from her broken slumber by a phone call at 2 a.m. with instructions on where to meet us in town. She never complained about this and said she'd rather see us all home safe. It would always result in my friends telling me I have the nicest mum ever. Which is true, as Grandma is always nice to everyone she meets.

After Uncle Matthew and I started school and didn't need her around as much, she took on the job which would see her through to retirement. Once we Hodges find something we like we tend to stick with it! She became a school secretary at a Church in Wales school in Llandaff. Llandaff is a lovely little 'city within a city', just a mile or two out of the centre of Cardiff, and is home to the beautiful Llandaff Cathedral. Grandma loved working in the admin office at the school with her bright, bubbly and beautiful friend, Heather. Their office formed a central hub of the school where pupils and teachers alike would pop in if they wanted cheering up, a chat or a lovely cup of tea. They pretty much had to shove her out of the door when it came to retirement, as I think she'd have happily carried on working there for ever!

I've already told you about Grandma being a big worrier and that probably my anxiety is a hereditary thing handed down through the female generations on her side of the family. But whereas I see it as something to be dealt with, managed and challenged, Grandma will bat away offers of CBT, meditation and talking therapies, and say 'it's just the way I am'. She's worried and catastrophized for so long I think it is almost a comforting feeling for her now. But that doesn't mean that I can't challenge her! You'll remember in the last chapter, Freddie, I told you how all of our family holidays were spent in the UK as Grandma would never get on a plane? Well, all the foreign holidays I went on in my teens and twenties must have softened her 'no-fly zone' attitude just enough for her to casually mention one day that perhaps she might get on a plane for her sixtieth birthday. Well, no sooner had the words come out of her mouth than I was on the computer booking three flights to Rome and there was no turning back! When you've been waiting for a long time for something to happen, Freddie, you need to seize the day while you can!

I'd decided to book us onto British Airways in the hope of it being a more pleasant experience for her than fighting for a seat on a budget airline. We told one of the air stewardesses, Juliet – Grandma remembers her name even now as she was so nice to her – that it was her first flight and she was very nervous. Juliet calmed her nerves and promised to check in on her during the flight. So I spent the next half an hour or so of the whole take-off process with Grandma's clammy hand tightly clutching mine like some sort of nervous jailer. She mostly sat there with her head down and eyes firmly shut – apart from whenever there was a noise and she would look up at me quickly in terror. It went a bit like this … Whoosh – terrified look – 'it's just the plane taking off' – head back down. Clunk Clunk – terrified look – 'wheels coming up' – head back down. Whirr whirr – terrified look – 'wing-flaps helping to steer plane right way' … You get the drift! Once we were up and cruising, though, she actually managed to relax and enjoy it a bit just as the lovely Juliet came back and slipped us three little bottles of champagne 'to celebrate Mum's first flight'. Grandma still has those bottles in her display cabinet at home. A historic moment!

There followed a fabulous few nights where Grandma, Grandad and I saw all the sights of Rome, ate our own body weights in pasta and pizza, and sampled the odd pot of gelato as well. I've been on many a holiday with Grandma and Grandad as an adult. I know not everyone would choose their parents as holiday companions, but I genuinely enjoyed spending time with them and we always had such lovely trips together.

Grandma is a huge armchair sports fan. She never takes part in any sport, but always likes to watch from the sidelines. She is a massive Formula 1 fan and loves the tennis, cricket, rugby, athletics and swimming. You name it, she'll be watching it. I think she might even watch more sport than your daddy, Freddie, though I'm not sure that's even possible! Sometimes she will take it from the armchair to the ground or track and we've spent some lovely trips going to various F1 races around Europe, watching the cricket at Glamorgan's ground in Sophia Gardens and of course our favourite – sipping champagne on Centre Court at Wimbledon. We love the atmosphere there and the beautiful surroundings of SW19 with its flowers in full bloom and courts so lush and green.

The other thing Grandma loves is a chat! She has struggled with loneliness since your grandad died, as a huge personality like his – with all the accompanying noises I've mentioned and will revisit shortly – will leave a huge void in a home. But I'm really proud of the way she has built up new friendships with people and found lots of things to keep her occupied. I've always tried to call or Facetime her every night so she doesn't sit through whole evenings alone. Before I know it we'll have been chatting for an hour about what's been happening over the previous twenty-four! And when I come to wrap up and say goodbye, she will say goodbye and then carry on chatting for another five minutes as more things pop into her head that she hasn't yet told me!

I had always envisaged me doing that with you as I got older, 'Just one more thing, Fred …', until you had to gently hang up on me to shut me up. For even speaking to you now, just as you are able to hold simple conversations, is a joy and a wonder. I'm so sorry that I will miss out on all those proper chats with you when you're all grown up, Freddie. But perhaps we can pretend and when you feel you need to tell me about your day, or anything that's going on in your life, picture me with you and I will do my best to answer everything you need to know.

* * *

Grandad Hodges, my dad, left us in July 2014 after a particularly brutal battle with oesophageal cancer. But let's not define him by his cancer as I hope I won't be defined by mine when I am gone. We'll go back to the beginning instead to when David James Hodges was born in October 1944, just before the end of the war, to Muriel and Robert Hodges. This timing gave him one of his favourite and most oft-used phrases, 'I'm a war baby, I am', which he used to explain his habit of not letting anything go to waste, be that food or the little bits and bobs he kept in jars in the garage 'just in case' they came in handy again (they rarely did!). He always took great delight in telling the story of how his mum went into the butcher's one time to use her meat coupons. She turned her back on him for just a moment and looked back to see him chomping away on a black pudding that she then had to use her precious coupons to buy! Grandad's mum and dad were Londoners from Plumstead way. I still remember my granny calling me 'duckie' like a proper London granny. My grandad didn't fight in the war as he had a protected-status job in Post Office Telephones as an electrical draughtsman. They had my Auntie Marion first in 1939, followed by my Uncle Bob in 1943 and by the time your grandad was born in 1944 they had moved to Gloucester. Your great-grandad was transferred to Wales when grandad was five. They moved into the little terrace house in Penarth that I remember visiting as a child, and eating their fish and crinkle-cut chips.

So, your grandad Hodges was English by blood but Welsh by heart. In his later years, if anyone accused him of being an Englishman abroad he could tell them he'd lived in Wales longer than most Welsh people! He certainly spoke with the accent and supported Wales in the rugby as passionately as the most red-blooded of Welshmen. He loved a pint down his local, the Dynevor Arms, where he'd sit amiably arguing with his group of friends down there. Now Grandad had a great sense of humour – I think it's where I get mine from, though I like to think my humour is somewhat more refined – but he also had an encyclopaedic memory for God-awful jokes. And he'd trot them all out as often as he could! His friends at the pub would have a similar reaction to me, a bit of an eyeroll and let the tumbleweed blow through as we'd heard them all so many times. But occasionally he'd find a new audience and a joke would land. Uncle Matthews friends were frequently fertile ground for this, so much so it was they who christened him 'Dave and his one-liners'. Then he'd be in his element firing out 'grandad jokes' like a World War Two soldier firing a machine gun:

'I used to be a werewolf, but I'm okay noooooowwwwww …'

'What's that *upside-down crab-hand gesture*? I don't know either, but here comes another one!'

'How do you tell the difference between a stoat and a weasel? A weasel is weaselly distinguished, when a stoat is stoatally different.'

'Stop that! Certainly, which way did it go?'

These were then generally followed by some sort of noise from Grandad's sound repertoire that he like to intersplice with the jokes. There was the foghorn – 'Arrrooooooggahh' – or often the pig (which always perplexed your daddy somewhat) – 'Oink!' – which he would use almost as a punctuation point in conversations. Though I think Grandad wasn't always aware of the noises he was emanating. Whenever he was in a high state of concentration he would hum loudly and unmelodically in a tone that would resonate throughout the house, but if one of us called from another room for him to shut up, he'd always be 'Shut what?!' But we always knew a humming daddy was one happily ensconced in what he was doing. As he would have said, he was 'like the proverbial pig in poo'!

Grandad loved music but as I told you earlier he was completely tone-deaf. When his friends put together a band when they were teenagers he really wanted to be in it, but couldn't sing or play any musical instruments – a bit of a hindrance. So he became their manager and drove them to their gigs instead! Around the same time, he met Andy Fairweather Low, who went on to play in the sixties band Amen Corner, and later would proudly recount his memories of hanging out with the future star. I'm not sure Andy F-L would remember him, but he certainly made quite the impression on your grandad! And I always recall being very proud to be able to take him to a special gig Andy put on when I worked at the BBC in Swindon, one of the first times he was really impressed by my job!

Despite his lack of discernible musical talent I remember all those car journeys on holiday when we were young as Grandad introduced us to his eclectic musical repertoire and left me with a lifelong love of sixties music in particular. There was everything from Chuck Berry, the Beatles, Bob Dylan, the Carpenters and Don McLean to the Everly Brothers, the Beach Boys, John Denver, the Rolling Stones and Elkie Brooks! All delivered via the top-quality cassette player in the Sierra. He always hankered after being a guitarist, forever fascinated to see the different instruments guitarists used up close. The engineer in him was always better at taking them apart than playing them effectively, but that didn't quash his enjoyment one bit. By the time he died he'd amassed a collection of six guitars, plus one ukulele (an inspired gift from me, I think) which seems a lot for a man who couldn't really play. But they gave him a lot of pleasure and you can learn from Grandad Hodges here, Fred, that just because you may not be the most talented at something it doesn't mean you can't enjoy it just as much as the next man!

* * *

Grandad had always idolized his older brother, Robert, my Uncle Bob. Just a year and a half apart in age, Uncle Bobby was that little bit taller than Grandad and from all the pictures I remember seeing of him – I think Grandad would have agreed – a little bit more dashing. They were the best of friends and loved spending time together. They both joined the Air Cadets in Penarth and both wanted to go on to join the Royal Air Force. Uncle Bobby did, but Grandad with his glasses was turned down because his eyesight wasn't 100 per cent and therefore not good enough to be a pilot. And he only wanted to be a pilot.

When Uncle Bob was killed on 27 December 1979 in an RAF Puma helicopter crash in Rhodesia, Grandad was crushed. Bob left behind my lovely Auntie Myra and my cousins Lorraine and Robbie, who were eleven and four at the time. I don't have any real memories of Uncle Bobby because I wasn't yet two when he died, but I remember a set of post-Christmas pictures of Grandad sitting with Uncle Matthew and me on his knees on the living-room chair, wearing a black jumper and tie, with red-rimmed eyes full of pain and sorrow.

Uncle Bob had been posted to Rhodesia at a time when British forces were monitoring events leading up to the country's transition from Rhodesia to the Republic of Zimbabwe. He was flying water-purifying equipment to the north of the country when the helicopter blades touched very high telegraph wires while following a road. The Puma crashed and the crew died instantly. Uncle Bob, who was the master air loadmaster, was thirty-six. The two pilot officers were just twenty-three and twenty-five. Losing his wonderful big brother was not something Grandad talked about much over the years, as I think it was just too painful for him. But before he died he managed a trip to the National Memorial Arboretum in Staffordshire to see Uncle Bob's name on the war memorial there. I sometimes think, or perhaps hope, that one of the people that Grandad seemed to be able to see around him as he was dying was Uncle Bob. There was a moment, as he stared into the empty corner of the room, when he acknowledged someone he could see there with such a warm beatific smile that spread across his face, one of recognition and love. It had to be Uncle Bob. Whether it's just a hallucination created by a dying brain or our loved ones really do come to take us to the 'other side', it gave me some peace to see that moment of happiness. Even in the seemingly worst situations in life, my Fred, there are some positives to be found if you look hard enough for them.

* * *

Grandad Hodges worked as a salesman in various guises, but he was very much of the 'work to live' brigade and enjoyed his time out of the office way more than in it. Uncle Matthew was a member of the Cubs in primary school, before graduating on to the Scouts. The Scout group was run by a friend of Grandad's called Rhod, who needed an extra adult supervisor to join them on their annual summer Scout camp every year. Grandad leapt at the chance, unlike your mummy, Fred, who likes a nice air-conditioned hotel room with plump pillows and a lovely view. My dad was never happier than when rolled up in his sleeping bag with a giant, plastic, orange bivvy bag wrapped around it, like some sort of ginormous sweet. If the weather was slightly damp and the tent a bit snug then so much the better! He'd be the happiest one getting on the bus in the centre of Creigiau, as all the boys waved goodbye to their families for the week, and one of the saddest getting off, as his week of scouting fun was over. But on his return home he'd always be enormously thrilled to see whichever was number-one golden retriever at that time and also Grandma, who he'd always jokingly refer to as 'the current Mrs Hodges'! His chief job on these Scout camps was cook, which is bizarre as he did very little cooking at home. But those Scouts must have had strong stomachs as they would make it through the week fuelled by the sausages, bacon and eggs that Grandad would fry up in industrial quantities for them.

We'll get on to Grandad's amazing mending and fixing skills shortly, but alongside those talents he loved to whittle wood, sit by campfires and lark around in the water with canoes and kayaks. It's like he was born to be a Boy Scout. So, as he began to head towards retirement he went on lots of training courses and joined the 1st Creigiau Scout Group Committee. He was treasurer for a few years before he got his big break and the chance to be Group Scout Leader, which he did for three years until he died. He helped to make improvements to the lovely little Scout Hut facility they have down by the woods and stream at the edge of the village. And he was to be found there on many an afternoon or evening with his mate and fellow Scout leader, Paul, giggling away like schoolboys.

I feel like in that Scout group he'd found somewhere he could really be himself – a big kid! Some of the warmest and truest words we heard about him at the funeral were from his scouting friends, who all wore their full uniforms in his honour. One of my favourite stories, which I learnt from William at the Scouts in the days after Grandad died, was the moment he had commanded silence on the minibus as it drove through Wiltshire on the way to another Scout camp. This was back in the days before digital radio and online streaming, so you could only hear the local stations when in the area. Grandad apparently shouted for all the Scouts and leaders on the minibus to stay silent on pain of death: 'I want to hear my baby on the radio!' The troop members were duly forced to listen to my news bulletin about the latest Wiltshire goings-on, before Grandad said, 'She's pretty good, isn't she?' and the journey carried on. The remembrance teddy bear we had made for you from his clothes while I was pregnant is crafted using much of his scouting clothing and proudly bears its own little yellow neckerchief and woggle. Shipshape, just as Grandad would have wanted. I always thought the scouting movement was a great institution, Freddie, especially now they've opened it up to both sexes instead of keeping it just for boys. It is something I would love for Daddy and you to get into together someday, if you feel it interests you. I think the combination of fresh air, making friends and doing lots of activities is perfect for busy little boys who never stop moving!

* * *

Another of Grandad's great loves in his later life were the Freemasons. Now the Masons have had a pretty bad rap over the years, as people don't like it when you won't tell them your secrets! But from what I could see from the few functions I went to, it's an older gentlemen's dining club that gives a lot of money to charity. Always one for a social occasion and a fancy uniform, Grandad was hooked. His main lodge was the Lodge of Concord in Cardiff, but he was also a member of a number of others, including one of the same name in Southampton. There's a fair old bit of regalia involved, with different types of small white apron worn over a dinner suit. Some were really quite ornate and valuable. Grandad was often to be found in the kitchen polishing them up (don't ask) and – you guessed it – humming!

In his later years, Grandad Hodges was also a member of the Pentyrch Bowls Club in the neighbouring village, as well as being part of the crib team in Creigiau Golf Club. As I mentioned in an earlier chapter, he was a member of the Creigiau 23 men's dining and charity-raising club for years and was its longest-serving member until he died. He was a busy bee, your Grandad Hodges. I can't think where you and I get it from!

* * *

Grandad was the early adopter of the Barbour and wellies, and loved stomping up and down the old disused railway line with whoever the current Hodges retriever happened to be. He loved to fix things, so perhaps you've also inherited your love of tools and mending things from him as well as your grumpiness. He was actually the best with a needle and thread in our house as Grandma had never really learnt and the war baby in him meant he'd often be the one fixing my riding jackets and bits of horse tack. In fact his ancient old Barbour jacket that he'd splashed out on in Harrods on our first family trip to London together became a bit of a 'Trigger's broom' (Google it!), so many times had it been patched up and lovingly stitched back together. A lot of those 'humming' moments happened while he was sat happily in the kitchen putting dubbing wax on our jackets and riding boots.

There wasn't anything that Grandad wouldn't have a go at fixing. Whenever he came to visit me after I left home there would always be a list of things to be hung, screwed into place or fixed as long as your arm. He was also number-one removals guy, so every time I moved he would turn up in a white van and dutifully help me pack up all my furniture and worldly goods, load it onto the van and then unload it all on the other side. As I mostly lived in first-floor flats you'll understand that this involved a lot of lugging heavy stuff up and down stairs. But he never once complained or didn't want to help, his only payment being a cold beer and curry at the end of it.

When I lived in a flat in Bristol and ordered an Ikea sofa that was probably a touch too big to get up the stairwell, it was Grandad who came up with a way of getting it around the corner and commanded his delivery-men troops like the best general from the landing. This was shortly followed by another issue with the same sofa not getting through the tiny L-shaped hall and into the lounge of my next flat in Swindon – it really was a very big sofa. So, never one to be defied by the laws of simple physics, Grandad set about sawing through the top of the wooden door frame, carefully removing the glass skylight pane so he could source another identical piece of glass and bam, the sofa was in place! Grandad returned a week later with his tools, wood and the new glass, and the door frame was as good as new, in fact probably better than when it was built the first time. I think he was very glad when I stayed in that flat for a good five years so as not to go through the stress of moving his daughter and her oversized items of furniture again.

My time in Swindon coincided with when Grandad's job as a sales rep happened to find him covering that area of the UK. It meant he was able to use his hotel allowance to stay at Chez Daughter and we'd always go out for a curry together to our favourite restaurant just round the corner called Biplob. We'd share enough food to feed about three times our number and put the world to rights over the 'chicken jalfrezi' – me – and 'something really hot with lamb' – Grandad. We also went on a few trips to see the Formula 1 motor racing, just the two of us.

When I decided, aged eighteen, that I really wanted to go and watch motor racing up close and threatened to book a trip to Spa-Francorchamps in Belgium (the cheapest foreign option on the motor-racing circuit at the time!) on my own, Grandad stepped up to come along with me. I'd got all the kit together for hiking around the hilly circuit at Spa before we went, including earplugs for both of us, to lessen the sound of the ear-splitting screams of the F1 engines as they tore around the track. Grandad had casually tossed his pair into the backpack before we'd set off for the circuit, with a 'Nah, won't need them'. I cried with laughter as the cars roared out on their first practice run, sending him diving into said rucksack and shoving the little orange wedges of foam into his ears before he gave himself tinnitus.

We stayed in the centre of Brussels between track days and it's where Grandad first introduced me to the delights of mussels and chips, which would become our go-to meal when I eventually moved from Swindon to London. There was a great little chain of restaurants called Belgo that almost exclusively sold mussels and chips with a Belgian beer menu the size of *War and Peace*. Ten or more years on from that first trip to the F1 at Spa, I was able to return the favour and babysit

Grandad a little while after he had his heart attack and had still insisted on going to Spa, leaving Grandma in paroxysms of fear. I really didn't take much persuading when a free F1 trip was on offer, but I did a great job in the role of nurse by stopping him from stomping up and down the hills at too fast a pace and getting him to rest for a while every time he looked out of breath.

As it turned out, the weak heart wouldn't be the thing that killed your Grandad Hodges, it would be that infernal cancer. He started having difficulties with swallowing late in 2012 and it turns out the years of indigestion and acid reflux he'd suffered – he was always popping an Alka-Seltzer or two – had turned into something called Barrett's oesophagus, where the damage from the reflux turns cells in the gullet abnormal, which can lead to cancer of the oesophagus. If these pre-cancerous cells are picked up early they can be treated, but of course Grandad was one of those men who never felt the need to trouble the doctor about his indigestion and therein was his undoing. Never be afraid to visit a medical professional about any health issue, Freddie. At the very least they'll send you away full of relief at good news; at the very worst, if there's something that needs fixing, then the quicker it's done the better.

By the time Grandad's swallowing issues were addressed he already had quite a significant tumour blocking his oesophagus. He started on chemotherapy to shrink it, which had great success with the tumour disappearing on scans. Then he had to make the choice of whether to have a massive operation called an oesophagectomy to remove any cells left behind. This, remember, was in the lead-up to our wedding and he was desperate to walk me down the aisle. Grandad, being a belt-and-braces kind of guy, opted for the big op. He'd already lost a lot of weight through being unable to eat in the build-up, but he worked as hard as he could to be in the best shape for our wedding day. As I told you earlier, he carried out his duties with aplomb, but we knew he wasn't the Grandad of old as he retired from the party early to go and rest. My well-covered, ruddy-cheeked daddy would have been leaping around like a loon with us to 'Mr Brightside', no idea of what he was dancing to, probably throwing in multiple foghorns and having a rip-roaring time doing it.

Grandad's cancer returned and he died with Grandma, Uncle Matthew and me at his bedside, holding his hands as he took his last breath on 1 July 2014. His funeral was hugely well attended with many packed in and standing at the back. He was brought into the crematorium to the strains of the Beatles' 'In My Life' and we left to another of his favourite Beatles tracks, the beautiful 'I'll Follow the Sun'. Our childhood vicar Father Graham, who by then was a Canon at Llandaff Cathedral, took the service. There were eulogies from his friend and fellow Scout leader, William, who had us in stitches with some of his memories of Grandad on Scout camp. Uncle Matthew spoke about his relationship with Grandad. And I talked about my daddy, something I'd toyed with as an idea from the moment I knew his cancer was terminal. Does that sound a familiar concept here, Fred? This is what I wrote and said about him on the final day of goodbye:

If my dad was here with us today ... he would probably have made a tasteless joke by now about this crematorium being the 'dead centre of town' ... or he'd be making some quip along the lines of ... 'I told you I was ill!' Famed for his one-liners and sometimes dodgy sense of humour, I'd often berate people, particularly my husband, Steve, for laughing at his jokes. I warned him they may be funny the first time you heard them but after thirty-six years they wore a little thin. But that was my dad, a big kid who was full of fun. One of my favourite pictures of him was taken just before he got ill, as he came with Steve and I to collect our new puppy from Carmarthen. We bought him from the same breeder as Mum and Dad had got their dog Tilly – who also joined us for the trip. The breeder rolled her eyes at Dad's lead control as the pair of them ran giddily through the field next door – Dad following the dog, arms outstretched aeroplane style. Dad was making people laugh right up to the end … just a few hours before he died, one of the nurses had a wry chuckle as she spotted the tot of whiskey that had been marked up on his medicine chart a couple of days before.

But Dad wasn't just a failed comedian. He was my man with a van. My Mr Fix-it. My numbers guy. If I needed shelves putting up, Dad was there the next weekend. If I wanted endless Ikea furniture putting together – Dad never grumbled. When I asked for a hand holder to accompany me to court on a speeding ticket (and pay the fine!) Dad took the day off work to be at my side. My first triathlon – Dad drove two hours up the M4 to carry my bike. The time I threatened at eighteen to go to my first Grand Prix on my own … Dad completely selflessly … offered to accompany me. I of course returned the favour by looking after him at his first Grand Prix after his heart attack six years ago. He kept the books for my company and went to London instead of me for the yearly meeting with my accountants. Dad was a doer – the most practical of men.

His skills were best put to use when, quite stupidly, he agreed to buy me a pony when I was thirteen. Previously knowing nothing about horses, Dad turned his hand to converting outbuildings to stables, mucking out, grooming and feeding. Dad was an early riser and I've never been a morning person so all of this was generally on the early shift before work. But Dad never complained and in fact loved it so much that at the ripe old age of fifty, he decided perhaps he should learn to ride too. Not long after Dad got his own horse ... his beloved Welsh cob Rhys. Dad and I would then go off to shows together, dressed in our smart black jackets and stock ties. I would enter all the showjumping classes. Dad would enter ... nothing. He was perfectly happy just to swan around the showground, looking the part and getting compliments on what a fine and handsome beast his horse was.

But my most happy memory of Dad will be as he walked me down the aisle to marry Steve last September. I am so glad we have that day to look back on and that he got to do his most important Daddy duty for me. He'd had one of the biggest operations a man can possibly have – just three months before. But his doctors were under no illusions that he absolutely had to be fixed by September the 14th. And he did it. It must have been such a long day for him ... he was up early to get ready and drink a whiskey with my husband-to-be. He tied the best tie knot of all the men in the wedding party. He sat without moaning – waiting for me to get ready – as (for those of you who weren't there) I was a touch late. And despite not knowing where he'd get the energy, he delivered what was described by one of my friends a couple of days ago as 'the BEST of dads speeches'.

My dear Daddy ... I was so proud of you then and I am so proud of you now. I like to think you're up there somewhere ... with your guitar in hand, the amp turned up to ten and telling some faintly vulgar jokes. I will miss you Daddy, every second of every minute of every day until we meet again. And always know Daddy – that I love you so very, very much.

* * *

The thing I heard most from teachers throughout my school years were that my brother, your Uncle Matthew, and I were like 'chalk and cheese'. I was studious, worked hard and got good grades. Uncle

Matthew messed about, rarely listened to what he was told, yet still, annoyingly, received pretty good marks. One of his primary-school teachers told Grandma and Grandad one parents' evening that he was most frustrating as she'd see him mucking around at the back of class, ask him what she'd just been saying and he'd repeat it straight back to her! He's very clever, your Uncle Matthew, and if he'd just apply himself he could achieve great things … now I feel like one of his teachers.

We were both into completely opposing subjects. I was the creative who loved English, history and drama but struggled with maths and sciences. He was the engineer, great at maths, physics and computing. Even now he will wax lyrical about some computer work he's doing or games that he's playing and it will all whizz straight over my head. Likewise when he starts talking about his beloved car! He's a bit of a boy racer at heart and before his girlfriend, Kirsty, came to sort him out and dig him out of his bachelor den, he could be found most evenings on the full-size car-racing seat he'd bought to race against friends on different circuits on the TV in his living room. Another Peter Pan who refused to grow up. If you ever need any help with cars or computers then he is your guy, my Freddie. If you want emotional and pastoral support, then you'll need to look elsewhere!

Even though we fought like cats and dogs when we were younger, as we grew up we actually became friends and used to hang out together. Whenever we went 'out to town' in Cardiff, if I decided to leave early – and I often would when I'd had enough, as I was a bit like a homing pigeon – Uncle Matthew would always come out to find a cab with me and then take down its number plate and make me promise to call as soon as I was home safely.

Uncle Matthew had your cousins, Emily and William, with his then wife, Gemma, before they separated. I think he actually became a better father because of it as he was forced to be more hands-on during the two days a week that he would see them. You see, Uncle Matthew totally has a heart of gold, but he doesn't always notice other people's emotional needs until they're shouted in his face! And that is what is so wonderful about his current partner, Kirsty – she totally 'gets' him. And she's the only one of us who knows how to control him! She's like the 'Matthew Whisperer' and I'm so very glad that she came into our lives when she did to restore a little bit of calm and whip your uncle into shape. One less thing for me to worry about … two, in fact, as she's brilliant with Grandma as well, a real fairy godmother. I hope she stays for ever.

Chapter 12

ALL CREATURES GREAT AND SMALL

I've always thought you can tell a lot about people based on how they treat their animals, Fred. Those who can show genuine love and affection for their pets and animals tend to be good. Always be very wary of those who are unkind to any of the beautiful creatures we are lucky enough to have on this planet. I hope you will always be gentle and kind to animals, Freddie. I see that wonderful bond you have with Bodie and at the moment we are just trying to teach you the difference between a gentle loving cuddle for him and one that is perhaps a little too aggressive! But these are nuances you need to learn as a toddler.

When I was born, your grandparents didn't have any animals and they'd never really thought about getting a pet. Guess who persuaded them? Yep, it was Mummy. Turns out I had them wrapped around my finger from the age of five! Our next-door neighbours had a golden retriever called Kerry who I was obsessed with. I used to go and knock on their door on a daily basis to ask if Kerry could come to play. So when they told us that she was having puppies and asked if we'd want one, the answer was immediately, 'Yes'! Well, from me anyway – it may have taken Grandma and Grandad longer to catch up but I was a done deal.

And so the first of the Hodges' golden retrievers came to live with us and Sophie was a lovely dog. I quickly learnt that owning a pet is not all fun when she chewed my brand-new M&S Girl sandals with a little heel that I was totally in love with, literally on the day I got them – there were a lot of tears from me! Then your grandparents got their first lessons in the ups and downs of pet ownership when Sophie chewed a big hole in the carpet in the hallway (that was fine by me – it was a pretty hideous seventies striped-orange affair and in need of changing!). A few nights later, when Grandad's boss had come for dinner, Sophie decided to pee on the lounge carpet right in front of him. It was not a high point. But no matter what she chewed and peed on, we all loved her. When she was tiny, Grandad used to tuck her into the inside pocket of his Barbour and take her down the pub for a pint, where she was always the star attraction.

Sophie lived to the grand old age of thirteen, so was part of the fixtures and fittings as we grew up. Grandma and Grandad wanted a bit longer to grieve for her, but as the school holidays were just around the corner it was a perfect time to be training a new puppy, with Grandma off work for six weeks. So I managed to persuade them that it was a good time to get another dog or we'd be waiting another year to get one. You can see who was the driving force behind the Hodges family pets when we were younger! But boy they were glad. Katie came from a lovely couple in Ross-on-Wye and was bred from their family pet retriever. I always felt especially close to her as Grandad, Uncle Matthew and I collected her while Grandma was on the last few days of term and she sat on my lap in the car all the way home. It felt like such a privilege to be able to soothe this little ball of golden fluff and tell her she was going somewhere she'd be loved very much.

She was so sweet-natured and had such a soft mouth that she never once chewed up a toy. She still had the toybox full of teddies that I'd given her as a puppy right up until the day she died. She only lived to ten and I think your grandparents always felt robbed of more time with their beautiful girl. This time they were in full mourning and kept her beautiful little casket of ashes on 'her' chair in the lounge for quite a few months. You see, that's the other thing about having pets, Freddie – they help to teach you about life and death from a young age. For as humans live longer than most domesticated animals we have to deal with their deaths throughout our lives. I wish with all my heart that you could have just had the death of dear Bodie as your first experience of how unfair life can seem at times and how nothing in this life is guaranteed to last for ever. I so wish I could have been the one to nurse you through any periods of sorrow and I dearly wish mine had not been the first death you had to deal with.

You are still too young to understand the concepts of life and death and something not being there any more. You can't understand why the delivery man won't bring the parcel with your toy in it the moment we buy it, so I couldn't hope to explain right now why Mummy isn't here any more. Just know, my Freddie, that it is not because any of us did anything wrong or because I didn't try hard enough to beat my cancer – I did everything I could. But sometimes in life, like a dropped china cup that smashes into a thousand pieces, there are things that can't be fixed. And that can feel so so unfair, as I'm sure it will to you many times over the years. But life is not about fairness. Often the nicest people don't win and the most evil do. But as soon as you can accept that concept and get on with living life in the best way you can and with good intentions, then you will be making your mummy very proud.

After Katie, came the current Hodges retriever, Tilly. Like me and your Uncle Matthew at school, their personalities could at best be described as 'chalk and cheese'! In every way that Katie was soft, gentle and loving … Tilly was brusque, brash and bold. We always laughed that it was because she was brought up under a now retired Grandad's tutelage! She developed a habit of climbing up on the kitchen chairs, then onto the table and cleaning up the plates if we left the dinner things out and retired for a moment. She of course then got stuck, and couldn't make the big jump down onto the slippery floor, so would have to wait for one of us to hear her whines and come and rescue her. That last Christmas we spent with Grandad Hodges in our Alderley Edge house we heard a bit of post-dinner clinking and in horror we realized she was up on the table among our very expensive wedding crystal and china that was having its first run out. To be fair to her she didn't spill a drop from any of the glasses, but it was a tricky job extracting her from the pricey tableware. She was also a serial food thief with what Grandma would call 'twizzle paws' – all food would have to be pushed right to the very back of surfaces and even then with a bit of paw dexterity and determination she'd often manage to get to it. Tilly also has a very odd habit of eating tissues – whenever you see her diving for a bag and sleeve it's because she's used her Predator-like ability to track one down! She will bare her teeth if you touch her feet or try and drag her anywhere by her collar and she thinks she's the boss of everything! But you still love her.

Whenever she comes to stay you pay her way more attention than Bodie, you laugh when she snatches a biscuit from your hand – we always quickly count your fingers afterwards – and you don't even notice her snarls when we're trying to extract the pair of you from your 'aggressive cuddles'! The only thing is we sometimes forget she doesn't have Bodie-like levels of self-control and we leave sandwiches out where she can snatch them or worse, forget there are cows in the field next to the footpath … On a walk last summer, Grandma was persuaded to let Tilly off the lead in the fields – she doesn't have a brilliant recall when she sets her eyes on something, so Grandma often just walks her on the long lead. But persuade her we did and what a mistake that was! Tilly seemed to have run off ahead and we were all calling her (Grandma having already given her up for lost and dead) when I suddenly remembered 'THERE ARE COWS IN THE SIDE FIELD!' and what comes with every good field of cows? Yes, a LOT of cow poo. Cue Tilly appearing back on the path, never having looked more pleased with herself, covered – and I mean from ear tip to paw – in green, stinking cow poo. Just as we were about to head back to our beautiful home. Well, like I always say, if you don't laugh you'll cry, so after howling with laughter poor Grandma was consigned to the front driveway with the hosepipe – so the poo didn't get all over the garden you were playing in. A couple of bottles of shampoo down and she definitely smelled sweeter, but still had the colour of what Farrow & Ball might call 'Ogre's Halitosis'. Life lesson, Fred – dogs and cow poo are never a good combination.

Speaking about stinky dogs, I guess I should come back to our beautiful Bodie here, whose patience and virtues I waxed lyrical about in Chapter 9. Well, he is not immune to a bit of dirt either. He must know all the spots where the deepest murkiest bogs are on his trips out with the dog walker as he will find them every day without fail! Even this summer, after a 80°F+ day heatwave and drought he has been known to come back from a walk looking like he's been doing a bit of bog-snorkelling and stinking of bins. We do our best to hose him down in the garden, but at some point he has to come in. I think dog owners become 'nose blind' to the smell of their pets, but I'm pretty sure the waft of 'eau de stinky pooch' that hits people as they arrive at the front door must be pretty intense. But these are some of the trade-offs you have to make for the pleasure of unending love from a dog.

Whenever Daddy is lying on the floor with Bodie of an evening, breathing deeply into what we call his 'stinky ruff' of fur around his neck, he always exclaims how he never thought he could love an animal as much as he loves Bodie. But that is what animals do to you – they work their way into your heart very quickly and then never leave! We really lucked out with Bodie, who has always been so gentle, good and easy to train. He never once pooed in the house as a puppy and was toilet-trained within a fortnight. He passed all his puppy classes with flying colours. He's always had a brilliant recall and he doesn't tend to wander too far on a walk, otherwise who would throw his ball?

The other day you did your usual trick of picking at your breakfast and leaving most of your toast behind. We dashed out to see a friend and returned three hours later with that plate of toast still sat on the sofa. I even noticed a piece of it on the floor, surely dog territory by then, but it was totally untouched by doggy paw or face. What a good doggo, so he had the cold toast as his reward for patience. I sometimes think that of our two boys Bodie will be hardest hit in the short term after I die. He has already become my little shadow and will follow me around the house and sleep on the floor on my side of the bed. He will often sit and watch me anxiously of an evening. He has the most expressive eyes and face of any dog I've ever known and his brow will be slightly furrowed, giving an anxious set to those big brown eyes of his. If I ever get upset or cry about the latest bit of bad news around my treatment or when I'm not feeling well, he is there, dashing to my side, holding out his little paw and trying to lick my hand. In Bodie's simple world I think he believes a lick can cure anything – sadly, it's about as much use for curing cancer as the many crazy lotions, potions and natural cures that the emails and messages that bombard me tell me to try. So Bodie will also need an extra lot of big cuddles from his brother once I'm gone. He will be a sad little pup. Cuddle him tightly and bury your nose into his ruff for comfort just as your mummy has done a thousand times before you.

* * *

Horses naturally come next in the list of animals I'd like to bring home. I absolutely adored My Little Pony toys when I was young. Father Christmas brought me the stable one year and the princess castle the next! In case you're having trouble picturing toys of the eighties, these were little plastic ponies in all colours of the rainbow with manes and tails you could groom with one of their little brushes (again, this was before the brutal hairdressing phase kicked in). My first one, Cotton Candy, was pink with white spots on her bum. By the time I'd got fed up of them, I had enough plastic My Little Ponies to fill a ranch! I should also say that most of my knowledge of the workings and ways of ponies came from books I'd bought at school fairs, most of them written in the forties and fifties and with a very 'jolly hockey sticks' approach to horse ownership.

So my first experience of learning to ride came as a slight disappointment – it can best be described as chaotic. I went along with my friend to a nearby farm where she knew the daughters – who had loads of spare ponies knocking about that they would let us ride. Perfect! Not all of these horses and ponies were equally good though. My friend always bagged the pretty grey, Billy, who had a very comfy saddle and would do as he was told. I was excited about what my horse would be like ... As my friend urged her horse forward so I could get on the mounting block, I spotted my noble steed being led out of the stable and he was no Desert Orchid, God love him. Peanuts was a very shaggy-coated, little dun-coloured pony, with a slightly sagging back and a sullen glare in his eyes that said to me, 'I am the boss here'. I was able to see his slightly sagging back because HE DIDN'T HAVE A SADDLE. I enquired as to whether one might be necessary but was told no, there were none spare and he was easy to ride bareback. The other slight 'tack' issue we had was that the reins I was given to steer and perhaps stop him were not the leather kind that everyone else used. No, these were in fact made out of the orange baler twine used to tie hay bales. To be fair, they did do the same job, but my hands were rope-burned for weeks! Riding hats were tossed in a pile in the corner – you could grab whichever fitted, but none had straps. Riding-hat roulette!

We spent many a happy afternoon on the farm with one of the farmers' daughter, directing us around pretend gymkhanas and handing out old rosettes, like me with my toy My Little Ponies. I think Grandma began to worry about safety at some point, probably around the time I started mentioning jumping without a saddle. She swiftly booked me some more formal lessons at Pontcanna Riding School in Cardiff and bought me a top-of-the-range safety riding helmet. At Pontcanna there was a big seated area on one side of the covered riding arena, where she could sit out of the wind and rain and watch me ride, thinking her worrying days were over. Wrong.

Riding Peanuts bareback had really taught me how to stick on a horse when it was playing up. As my riding improved and I moved up the grades, I was quite often put on one of the 'fizzier' horses. There was one in particular called Brandy and if my name was up against his in the class list, Grandma would turn straight around, calling back, 'I'll be waiting in the car'! As he spent most of the lesson leaping around like he was fresh out of the Spanish Riding School of Vienna, on this occasion I think it was sensible.

You could go down to the riding school on weekends and evenings to help and I jumped at the chance to spend more time with the horses and learn how to look after them. It was my first experience of making friends outside of my village and school, and I have to say I found it perplexing. Riding schools can be cliquey places at the best of times and especially when you're shy. The group of kids who hung out there would sometimes just blank me for a day, and I had no idea why as I was too afraid to ask. I was very easily led and my forty-year-old feminist self now would have a stern word with her teenage pushover incarnation to speak up for herself. If you ever find yourself in this sort of situation, which I'm not sure you will as I can see you have much more confidence in yourself, then always ask the person who has an issue with you what it is and if you don't like the answer, move on. You don't need to be surrounded by people who aren't 100 per cent Team Bland! This is the place where I, trying my best to fit in, took up the dreaded smoking habit that would take me another twenty years to kick. Trying to fit in can be dangerous for your mental and physical well-being, my Freddie, so try to avoid being like someone else and concentrate on being the best version of you that you can be.

Once I was more confident completing the daily tasks needed to keep a pony fed and watered and happy, it was time to ask THE QUESTION. I sat your grandparents down and just came out with it straight ... 'Daddy, can I have a pony? PLEASE?' I nearly fainted in shock when my 'non-horsey, never ridden in their lives, no idea what's coming parents' said – 'Okay then'! What a moment, the one I'd been dreaming about for years.

Then we all looked at each other with the same thought. How on earth does one go about buying a horse? Remember, this was in the days before the Internet, where a quick search would have thrown up thousands of options within a five-mile radius. Luckily, Grandad knew a guy at the pub who knew a jockey called Phil, and that Phil could find us the perfect horse! It didn't take long before a suitable horse was brought to a stable in Hensol near Llantrisant for me to try out. She was a bay mare 14.2 hh (that's hands high – they still measure horses using an archaic system), part-Arab and with a little bit of Welsh Section D Cob and I fell in love the minute I saw her staring at me with her huge, incredibly intelligent brown eyes. She was a little 'green' and only just coming up for four years old, so not broken in very long. 'What's her name?' I asked, loads of regal options whizzing through my mind as a suitable moniker for this gorgeous horse. 'Uh yeah, we think she's called Craig?' What?! Craig? It would have to be changed. There was relief all round when we looked at her papers in which her full name was listed as 'Craig y Celliog Cariad', which roughly translates as 'the darling of cockerel rock'. The part used as her day-to-day name was Cariad – so beautiful and befitting of my new girl. Cariad simply means 'darling' or 'sweetheart' in Welsh and she was such a darling. That is when she wasn't being a bit of a bugger. We were very much made from the same stuff, me and Cariad.

After a few weeks of training we took her to her new home. Now this is a very forties pony-book solution. Our neighbours had a couple of stables in their garden that they were just using for storage and I'd asked if I could use one for Cariad. It meant I was on my own with her while I learnt the ropes of caring for a pony and it also involved walking her about a mile up the road to the field where she would graze. The straw that broke the camel's back on this complicated set-up was when she barged me out of the way at the stable door one day and ran out into the main road that leads through the village, her shoes making a panicky skittering sound as the metal hit the tarmac. And she was off. I quickly grabbed a lead collar and lead rope and charged after her. It was a twisty lane up to the field and then a very busy main road to cross. Luckily, a friend's mum picked me up as she was passing in her car and we raced after a now cantering Cariad, trying to stop her before she crossed the big 60 m.p.h. main road that ran adjacent to her field. Well, we didn't quite make it in time, but I cried tears of relief to see her standing by the gate to her field, ripping up big mouthfuls of the long green grass. Apart from being a bit sweaty and blowing like a train from her morning escapade, she was otherwise unharmed. I threw a lead rein and my arms around her neck and sobbed big fat tears into her coarse black mane. I felt at that moment that perhaps I wasn't very good at this pony-owning thing.

It was time for another 'Fix-it Dad to the rescue' moment. There was an ancient stone building at the bottom of the horses' field and Grandad asked the farmer if we could use it and section it off into stabling. Bearing in mind he was about ninety years old and a bit hard of hearing, we can never be sure how much he took in. But he seemed happy and so Grandad set about turning that stone shack into two little stables – one for Cariad and one for Sebastian, my new riding friend Gemma's little dapple-grey pony who also lived in the fields. A breeze-block wall was put up in no time at all and Grandad built two lockable stable doors out of some old wood into a V-shape at the front, so we could simply walk them out a few metres and release them into the fields for the day. No chance of any main-road racing here. We also had an old wooden shed which doubled as a makeshift tack room. It felt like we had all the mod cons! Grandad even managed to get electricity installed in the stables, so we could see what we were doing through the dark winter nights.

Gem and I would ride out in the fields, which were huge, and we put up a few little jumps in one. Cariad and Sebastian became inseparable and I finally began to think I was an old hand at this now. But pride comes before a fall, Freddie, and quite literally in this case. Cariad had developed a habit of 'bolting' – this is when the horse decides to take control and where the phrase 'take the bit between your teeth' comes from, I'd imagine. She would literally grab her bit – the metal part at the bottom of a bridle that sits on the horse's tongue and helps you to control it. In theory. Like I said, if she grabbed it with her teeth, put her head down low and galloped as fast as she could while I had no control over her, it was pretty scary! And if she decided to change direction too quickly then I'd be out of the side door and landing with a bang.

* * *

I should say at this point how incredibly generous and supportive Grandma and Grandad Hodges were of my riding endeavours because it is an expensive hobby. When I look at all the trips to the saddlery to buy bandages, boots for Cariad, boots for me, show jackets, new hats, stable rug for inside, New Zealand one for outside, they must have been shelling out a fortune every weekend and that's before you've even factored in stabling, food costs and the fees for entry into shows, classes, petrol and food on show days, and paying for a space on a horse lorry. The list goes on. But they made sure I was at every show I wanted to be at with all the gear and my usual no-idea! And they'd be clapping and cheering from the sidelines even though I was getting disqualified for three refusals at one fence!

That's exactly what happened at my first show at St Fagans. Nerves got the better of me and I wound myself up into a right tizzy. I spent most of the morning jumping huge jumps in the practice ring to make sure Cariad was up for the job that day. The course of jumps looked beautiful. I didn't think I'd win, but harboured hopes of a place in the top six so I could make the hack home with a beautiful rosette fluttering from Cariad's bridle. That was the plan. We trotted into the ring – me, resplendent in my smart, new, black show jacket and velvet-covered crash hat. Cariad's chesnut/brown coat was gleaming in the afternoon sun. I'd even made an attempt at plaiting her coarse black mane that of course was more cob than Arab.

The bell rang to signal I could start and I kicked her on into a canter as I circled round to the first fence. But something wasn't quite right. Instead of her usual lively, bouncy canter I got a tired, flat one and just as I pointed her towards the first fence, she dug her feet in like the stubborn mare she could be. Somewhat flustered and embarrassed, I circled her round and pointed her towards the fence again ... same thing. One more and we'd be out. So I circled her around one last time, valiantly aiming for the fence but losing all sense of riding style and skill, and we skidded into that first fence with Cariad's hooves clipping the bottom and knocking the fence poles to send them rolling everywhere. As if I couldn't have had a more ignominious exit from the ring, St Fagans was quite a large show, so as we trotted out of the ring, me red-faced and trying not to cry, the loud tannoy shared my shame with the whole show field: 'NUMBER 568 ... RACHAEL HODGES RIDING CRAIG Y CELLIOG CARIAD IS DISQUALIFIED FOR THREE REFUSALS AT THE FIRST FENCE.'

I learnt from this, that particularly where animals and children are involved, you can over-prepare and end up with them tired and grumpy. There's no shame in being disqualified in a sporting environment; at least you got up that morning and worked hard at something and TRIED. A lot of people don't bother to do that. As long as you can say you tried your best at something, Freddie, then that is all you can do. The more times you try, then the more likely you are to succeed. And don't be scared of failure, my Fred. It's those failures and how we react when things go wrong that shape who we are today. Failure can in fact make you a better, stronger, more resilient person.

* * *

After a few years Cariad did indeed become the great showjumper that I'd hoped she would be. Her prize-winning ways seemed to coincide with me getting better at riding – who'd have thought it? We'd moved her into a lovely livery yard just up the road, the kind of place that had proper stabling in barns, horses' nameplates on the stable doors, tack hung up neatly on hooks outside the stable. Grandad and I had settled into a great routine where he would do the early-morning muck-out and turnout – result! – and I would do the evenings after school, grabbing a quick ride if it was light enough and bringing Cariad into the stable to keep warm overnight. Cariad had the most impeccable stable manners. I could walk underneath her tummy to do up her night rug without her batting an eyelid. She would let you manhandle her around the box and she'd always be so gentle. Out and about, though, it was a different story. A proper Dr Jekyll and Mr Hyde pony. If something like a bit of rubbish in the hedge flapped in the wind she could go into meltdown and leap sideways across the road, often with no warning to me. Also very dangerous if cars are coming the other way. But I only ever had a few falls from her (thanks to all that clinging onto Peanuts with no saddle). Most were in the field and generally kids and teenagers just 'bounce' when they fall off their ponies – and remember, the smaller the pony the lower the centre of gravity!

It was inevitable that with all this work Grandad was doing to help look after my horse he might want to have a go at the fun bit himself. He was a little on the heavy side for my little Cariad, so at the grand old age of fifty he started going for riding lessons at Pontcanna Riding School himself! There, he'd always be put on the most enormous horse to fit a man of his size – I should point out he wasn't massive, just a little more weighty than their average clientele of skinny teenagers. Grandad was often paired with their fabulous part-shire horse Clyde – what a guy! – who measured in at a dizzying 18.2 hh. He took quite some riding around a small indoor school. Grandad's boss's daughter at the time had a fabulous Welsh Section D Cob called Rhys. She was off to university and got the idea in her head that she only wanted Grandad to ride and look after him (I'm not sure she'd seen him on one of his bad days with Clyde or she might have changed her mind!). So suddenly we were a two-horse family as Rhys joined our number. He was a fabulous beast of a horse at 15.2 hh, with a black shiny coat, flowing mane and tail and a huge crested neck. Grandad would take him to shows with me just to swan around on. He wasn't really interested in entering the classes, he just wanted to look the part and take in all the compliments about Rhys! The horse got so much attention and there were several offers to buy him. We actually bought him ourselves and the next few years were very happy ones filled with horses and Barbours and wellies!

However, that's not to say that as in life there weren't a few falls along the way. But you've just got to get straight back in the saddle. There was my harmless but rather hilarious fall at the Pentyrch show. In fact it's better to describe it as a drop rather than a fall. I was taking part in the pairs showjumping class, which is kind of a baton relay with two riders on each team. You need to race around a course of jumps as quick as lightning then hand over the baton, or more often a ribbon, to your partner and watch them tear around in record speed, you hope! Fastest time overall takes the silverware. Simple. Well, simple if you've tightened your girth beforehand. The girth is the strap that goes around the widest part of the horse's belly and needs to be tightened or loosened depending on how hard the horse is working. Some horses don't always co-operate fully with the doing-up bit and puff out their tummies as much as possible to keep the girth loose. Cariad was one of these.

After trying a few times I thought I'd just do it later, then of course managed to arrive at the pairs' jumping ring a little late with me and my partner Rebekah up next. She set off first, flew around the course clear, got back and tagged us in! We set off at the gallop and the jumps were only small so Cariad was pretty happy to take them at near full tilt. As well as speed, finding the shortest route around the jumps gets you to the end faster, so we were making sharp turns like the best of rodeo stars. Then I had a slight feeling I was off balance and slipping sideways, and I remembered the girth was on about as loose as it could be. Not wanting to stop and let Rebekah down, we carried on as fast as we could, with me and the saddle slipping further and further round. I took the last jump in ungainly fashion, using the reins to cling on (sorry Cariad!) and almost knocking down the poles with my body. Though we somehow made it over the finish line, Cariad skidded to a halt and deposited me right where I belonged, on the floor! There were a few sniggers in the crowd, which I'm sure would normally have deeply affected me at the time, but I didn't care as we had still managed to come in sixth place which meant we got a brightly coloured rosette to go home with! I'm THAT competitive I will keep going despite half falling off my horse. Sometimes, Freddie, while it may be easier to give up and take the fall, clinging on for dear life is a more satisfying option.

Grandad's big fall came in way more spectacular fashion – though no one was there to see it. He'd set off from the farm to ride on his own one day – I think I was now being a sulky teenager who didn't want to get up early and play ponies. The farm was at the top of a lane that steeply declined into a little hamlet called Rhiwsaeson then an almost 45-degree gradient to get near the top of the Caerau – a small (by Welsh mountain standards) hill that you could actually see from the top of Grandma and Grandad's road. You went through a gate on the left and into the grassy area around the top of the hill and Grandad and Rhys were making the most of their freedom and having a lovely canter, the breeze blowing in their hair. Well, Rhys's hair, as Grandad had very little by that stage. Grandad couldn't quite recall the sequence of events but as they were cantering merrily away, with him not paying full attention, Rhys spooked at something and dived one way, catching Grandad totally off balance, dispatching him, as we say in riding, 'out the side door'. He must have landed with quite some bash to his head because he was knocked out for a little while. He said he came to, sat on his bum in the mud on top of the hill – not remembering his own name – but thinking the year was around 1950 and he'd come off his motorbike! The ladies at the livery yard were quickly alerted to the fact there'd been a parting of ways between horse and rider after Rhys trotted back into the yard alone, trailing his reins behind him but with no David in sight. A search party was quickly dispatched and they met Grandad making his way unsteadily down the hill on foot, still not quite sure who or where he was!

We sold Rhys on when we were both riding less and as I went off to university. I could never bear the thought of actually selling Cariad – so I just didn't face up to it initially and let her go on loan (when you let someone ride your horse and they pay for stabling and look after it) to a woman at the yard. I eventually sold her on to Elaine, whose family owned the place, so I knew Cariad could stay in her home and be well looked after. She's now in happy retirement up there, outliving us all, and I've been to visit her a few times. Her beautiful lashes are now a little greyer and her bay coat not as glossy, but she's still my girl, my first – and only – pony.

After university I rode a few horses here and there on various holidays but never went back to riding in earnest. Then when I moved north from London to Cheshire, a very horsey part of the world, I became newly obsessed with buying a horse. There were lots of lovely livery yards around and some beautiful horses for sale. But then I began to remember what a drain on time and money horses could be and by then I had met your daddy and was thinking about a future little you before too long, and do you know what, Freddie? Mummy for once backed away from a pricey impulsive purchase! You could probably mark that point as the one I knew I really wanted to be your mummy as I needed to think about other people and not just myself.

Of course, I still wanted to get back in the saddle but none of the local riding schools seemed the right fit. Going round in a circle on a ploddy pony while having instructions shouted at me wasn't really my thing any more. But then I found a professional showjumping yard down the road and the owner James Davenport, an international showjumper himself, who could give me lessons on one of his horses stabled in the yard. Well, this sounded like my kind of place! We arrived at the electronic gates and drove in to see beautiful stables and a huge outdoor area with some pretty formidable-looking jumps set out. I met James and he showed me the horse I'd be riding. He was a handsome dark-brown stallion with very wise eyes and a fabulously soft velvety muzzle. Obviously such a prime specimen of horse power would go by a name like … Rambo. There was not a speck of dirt on his gleaming coat and tack, and I was a little overwhelmed by this dazzling place as Rambo gently clip-clopped out of the stables and into the yard. I got on via the mounting block as he was a good 17 hh of horse.

We set off behind James into the arena and wow – I could tell this horse was something special and not like one I had ever ridden before. We were criss-crossing the arena following James's orders to walk, trot and canter, and Rambo did it all on cue. It was the first time I'd been on a horse that had been trained to use the right 'aids' – the signals you give them to speed up, slow down and then stop. The gentlest nudge from my heel at his side and he'd be off into a canter, on the right leg. This had never happened to me before without a lot of kicking and cursing! Then when it came to head around the showjumps, which James had lowered significantly by this point, I might add, Rambo was just flawless. As the jumps went up the only thing that hindered him was my eye and trying to mess with his stride. I'd get terribly frustrated with myself but then James – a very calming presence with his soft Cheshire burr – would just tell me to bring him round the jumps again while he variously called out instructions to 'sit up', 'sit back' and 'just let him go'! I loved Rambo – I will never ride a horse as perfect for me as him again. So I was totally gutted to find out he'd been sold on to a lady in America – when I asked how much a horse like that would cost, it was in the tens of thousands. Way beyond my means. If I ever win the lottery it's been my dream to go over and see this American Rambo-stealing woman and ask her to name her price, though I'm told she would never sell him. She only competes in fairly novice events and there is always great interest in this beautiful, brown British steed. I have promised that I will go back and ride there again, though the cancer has kind of got in the way. But hey, the strapline on my blog says I'm 'Putting the can in cancer', so it's probably time I took my own advice and got back in the saddle.

I think you can probably tell, Freddie, by the amount I've gone on about it, that horses and riding are one of my happy places! If you don't fancy riding a horse yourself, and that's fair enough as it's not everyone's cup of tea, then think of Mummy every time you see horses when you're out and about. It's always a moment of true joy when we point out horses to you in fields and your little face lights up as you spot them too. Horses are our thing, my Fred – encouraging you to like them was one of the first times I felt I had some influence in your behaviour. I had hoped there'd be so many more and there still can be. Because that is why I am writing this book for you. I will still be present and central in your life and choices, within these pages.

Chapter 13

ADULTING

As I've said before in this book, Freddie, do NOT rush into being an adult. When you've finally reached the 'top adulting' status, the award you get in my head says, 'Well done, now you'll spend the rest of your life wishing you were young again'!

I guess my journey into adulthood started on that first day of moving into university halls in Cardiff. Considering I'd lived on the edge of the city all my life, it wasn't quite the bold break from home that many eighteen-year-olds strike out on, but the course I wanted to do was in Cardiff and it felt like the best of both worlds to live away from home but to be able to call your grandma over with a bag of shopping when money got tight! I had a lovely room in Talybont North Halls with a comfy bed, nice desk, shelves and my own little en-suite (much like sharing a bed, I'm not big on shared bathrooms!). I guess these days an estate agent might try and pass off this en-suite as a 'wet room' – it was totally plastic inside with no shower curtain. But all this would do Mummy just fine! I remember it as so new and fresh that it made me feel old when one of my next-door neighbours, a prospective student, went there to look round a couple of years back and declared it old and a bit tired … I suppose the intervening twenty years do that to all of us.

I always liked to take all my little creature comforts with me everywhere I moved to and once they were in place it felt immediately like home. Keepsakes and items you love can evoke very powerful and comforting feelings. I'd need my duvet cover that involved yellow, my books, my cheesy VHS film collection (ask your dad about VHS), pictures of friends and family, and a couple of posters bought from one of the freshers' events. I favoured Edvard Munch's painting *The Scream* because I thought it was a bit 'artsy' and the movie poster for a recent film I loved – Baz Luhrmann's *Romeo + Juliet*, starring a very young Leonardo DiCaprio and Claire Danes as the star-crossed lovers. I loved Claire Danes at this time as she'd just starred in the brilliant teen TV series *My So-Called Life*, which was sadly and inexplicably cancelled after just one season.

Creature comforts in place, things unpacked – my room felt like home, so now it was time to head out beyond the door and meet my new flatmates. I'd already met one – as I'd been lugging my stuff in downstairs my friend Julia, who I knew from school, shouted down. Once we did a bit of window counting we realized we were in the same flat! I headed back up, chuffed that I knew someone already and over the next couple of days the girls that would make my university life brilliant began to arrive before nervously emerging from their rooms one by one. There was Rach, with her West Country twang, foghorn laugh (she always got along with Grandad!) and wicked sense of humour. Tall, willowy Kathryn, a churchgoer, but not the shy and retiring kind, was also blessed with a loud laugh and sharp wit. There was Princess Sarah as we nicknamed her, always perfectly turned out, on top of things and a huge fan of Disney. I always imagined that when she went back into her room, she'd clean and dust in a Disney princess ballgown surrounded by little hummingbirds and animals of the forest! Then there was Julia, football fanatic, music fanatic, who liked nothing more than a night out involving both! And me, I didn't really know who I was at this stage, but what better place to find out than at university?

So there we were, like a budget version of the Spice Girls (very popular band at the time), ready to take on the next three years. Here are some valuable things I learnt at university:

1. If you only exist on Super Noodles, mini hotdogs, spaghetti on toast and all forms of brightly coloured alcohol YOU WILL GET FAT. I believe it's now called 'Fresher's Flab'.
2. A strategically placed poster on a wall can cover a multitude of sins, especially when you want your rent deposit back.
3. Once your student loan has run out, there is NO MORE MONEY. You may have to take some of your more rash purchases – when you were feeling rich – back to the store.
4. Credit cards are not free money, despite what their shiny, brightly coloured plastic will try to tell you. They will only make your financial situation worse.
5. Nothing good ever came of a night where alcohol is priced at less than a pound a drink. 'Eighties night' – you have a lot to answer for.
6. Nothing good comes of drinking games or alcohol races. If you're going to be drunk anyway, at least try and enjoy the drinking bit.
7. There is a bit of work and learning to do as well, but often this can be crammed into an end-of-term frenzy.
8. You will meet friends who you will have for life.
9. Just check they're not those annoying ones who post all your embarrassing pics straight on social media.

10. Tuition fees are expensive now, so remember you're there to learn as well as have fun!

I imagine things will have moved on a lot in the fifteen years between now and when you may go to uni. Perhaps you'll be doing all your modules remotely from a nice beach somewhere, logging into lectures and only drinking vitamin water. Or maybe you'll be getting drunk and dancing to cheesy pop on a sticky student-union dance floor just like we did. Whichever it is, I hope you have a lot of fun doing it.

* * *

When I look through our old uni pictures, as I did the other night when the girls came to visit me, it looks like aeons ago. We've become such close friends and I still can't believe twenty-two years have passed in the blink of an eye since we met. I have been Rachael's bridesmaid and she has been mine, and we've all been there for each other's weddings and expanded our number by ten and counting. Eighteen still seems very young and I'm not sure how we all survived being let loose on the world at that age. When I see a fresher moving in now, I just want to give them a hug and make them a cup of tea! But the other thing I see in the photos is how young and carefree we look. We are so happy and unburdened by real problems and I hope you can be like that, Freddie. To experience those happy times when the world is your oyster. (By the way, just for the record – I tried oysters once and they were, as you would say with a wrinkled-up nose, 'disgusting'.)

It wasn't all fun and games at university though. Trying to find somewhere to live after the first year of halls that wasn't absolutely stinking proved difficult. For our second year we took up residence in a mouldy palace on Malefant Street, right in the centre of students-ville in Cathays. This was the place I mentioned earlier in the book where I had a room with no windows. We always drew lots for our rooms and I always lost! Though poor Rach had to sleep in a front room that was full of mould and damp and did not do her asthma one bit of good. This was the place where we once found a slug in the fridge. I'll say no more.

The next year we thought we'd go up in the world with one of the professional landlords who owned a large number of student properties. You even got to pick your house from a price band – we went for the one below top, I mean we *were* students! Alas this one, though looking cleaner than the last one in that we didn't have to paint or stick posters over the damp, was probably worse. It had the world's most uncomfortable wooden-framed sofas, without enough seats for everyone. The cupboards all had curtains on them instead of doors which perplexed me no end. All of my shoes went mouldy in the bottom of the cupboard in my room, but I was told it was our fault for not having the heating on enough! Then came the army of mice. I thought I was pretty hardy. I never thought I'd be one of those girls to jump on a chair and scream when one appeared. Turns out I am that girl and the first time one came scuttling out from behind one of those damn cupboard curtains, trailing it behind like a superhero cape, I was up and on my chair screaming like the woman from the shower scene in *Psycho*! And I didn't even have the worst of it. One scuttled across the back of Rachael's bed in the night. In Sarah's room there was a hole in the floor through which one would just emerge, hoisting its fat little tummy though the tiny gap and scurrying off to try and steal some of her chocolate. After many pest controllers' visits, traps laid and chairs jumped on, we were told the mouse problem was actually coming from next door, which had been vacated by a family who'd left loads of junk behind. So as I recall we ended the mouse problem in the swiftest and easiest way possible – by moving out at the end of the year!

* * *

University was the first place I started to experiment with my 'look' and when I see the pictures again now I give an involuntary shudder. At the time I still had some of the insurance money left from my car crash and in my typical manner was frittering it away on some truly hideous clothes. I wish someone had pulled me to one side back then and said, 'Love, you're better off saving that money or investing it instead of trying to make yourself look like the sixth Spice Girl.'

I know this will be difficult for you coming from two spendthrift parents as you do, Fred, but when you come by money throughout your life, it's okay to buy one or two little treats but always try and save the rest, because having savings put away gives you options. And having options means freedom. What doesn't give you freedom is a wardrobe weighted down with eight of the same – well, differing putridly coloured – pairs of flared stretch trousers. From orange to red to fluorescent-green flowers I had a pair for every occasion! Then there was the stage of the see-through dresses with dragon appliqués on the front. If I'd ever had a daughter, she would have been sent straight back up to change if I saw her in one. I always went for the 'big pants' look underneath, but I'm not sure whether that helped or hindered the whole ensemble. This led me on to the tassled-dress period, before I got into a much more reasonable run of black Lycra or tailored dresses by my third year. My weight fluctuated somewhat at uni, which meant it was Russian roulette as to whether these hideous garments I've described would actually fit me. I put on that fresher's stone in the first year, then after a nasty comment from some careless boy over the summer I practically starved myself until I was a size 6. Then I met my university boyfriend Max and it started going up again with the 'happy new love' fat I talked about getting with your daddy earlier.

Max and I met while I was wearing my black see-through dragon dress, so I must have been on a thin period. I say 'met' – we'd already done that totally junior school move of getting my friends to tell his friends that I liked him, which was followed by him checking me out in the uni bar before we were thrown together for that nervous first chat at one of our friends' birthday parties. We both stood awkwardly by the bar, not knowing what to say. Friends are a safe ground aren't they, thought Max, and he opened with, 'So I think you know my friend, Jim?' Said 'Jim' had just messed with the heart of one of our girls and I was quite tigerish about it, so my deadpan reply was 'I do, and we all hate him in our house …' Good chat, Rach, good chat. That would need to be worked on. He can't have been too scared off, though, as we stayed together throughout university and beyond.

The other thing we need to discuss here is the state of my make-up back then. Teenage girls now look flawless to me with all the YouTube make-up tutorials you can watch these days. In fact they look so flawless it makes me sad that they'll have no tales of awful make-up to tell their children about! We were lucky back then to get any advice off the lady in Boots about whether we suited that sugar-pink shade of lipstick. The only brush I owned was a blusher brush – well, I used it for bronzer, which was the favourite back then. So my make-up consisted of heavily applied foundation, NOT in any way blended past the jawline. I didn't know what blending was back then or why you would do it with make-up! A bit of powder would be followed by a generous amount of bronzer, which would make me look as if my cheeks had been on holiday to Spain but the rest of me had not!

Then the eyeshadow. Oh, how I cringe at the eyeshadow. I favoured a bright green shade, applied using the sponge-on-stick applicator that came with it. This I piled on as thickly as possible in a half-moon shape above my eyelashes and along the lash line underneath. Then, and most importantly for this nineties look, NOT BLENDED! No softened edges, nada. I looked like Kermit the Frog. After some mascara – again liberally applied and lumping my eyelashes together – then it was time for the finishing touch. Loads of tiny sparkly jewels stuck down my cheeks. Just thinking about this make-up compared to what I wear today gives me an involuntary shudder. The worst bits were those little stick-on jewels which liked to wander off my face through the night, so as I hugged and kissed people hello I would notice I suddenly had several fewer, but then spot one of my friends across the bar with an erroneous sparkle about their visage. I usually just left them as a gift rather than have an awkward conversation about one of my jewels jumping ship!

I loved my course at university – Journalism, Film and Broadcasting – though still found it difficult to make friends with the other students. I feel this was a combination of my shyness and the 'resting bitch face' I had developed, which I just thought was a fairly passive face but turned out to be pretty unapproachable! If I could go back again I'd just try chatting with a few more people – it seems a pretty straightforward concept. Chat, get to know people, make plans together – boom – got friends. I hope you make friends more easily than your mummy, Fred. I feel like you will be more gregarious like your dad. As I watch you now, playing with other children, I can see you are confident and hold your own. And always remember you've nothing to lose by going and chatting with someone. They're probably feeling just as nervous as you and will welcome the interaction!

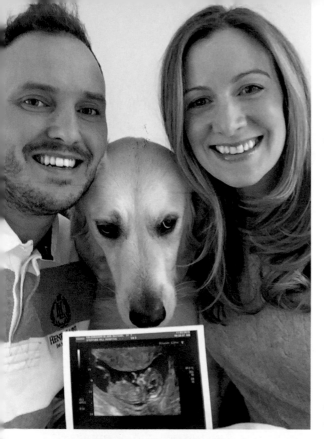

The first picture of you! Our twelve-week scan, beaming with joy. We couldn't wait to tell the world.

Your first nap after you entered the world. You were perfect.

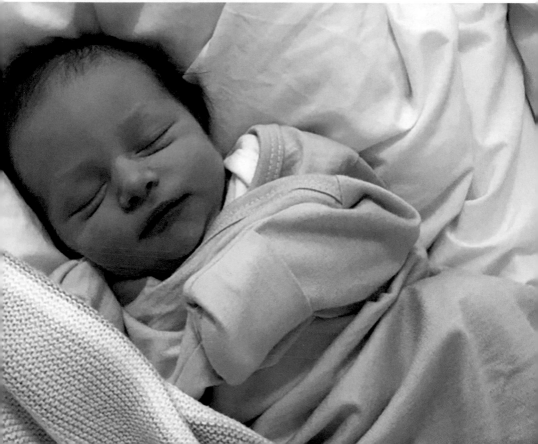

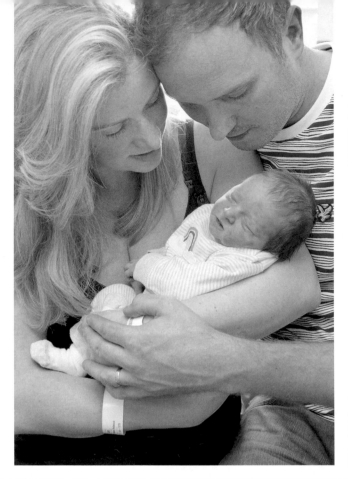

A snap taken just before we left the hospital to bring you home in September 2015. We couldn't stop looking at you.

With your Grandad Hodges's remembrance bear, made from his clothes. I know we will both be watching over you.

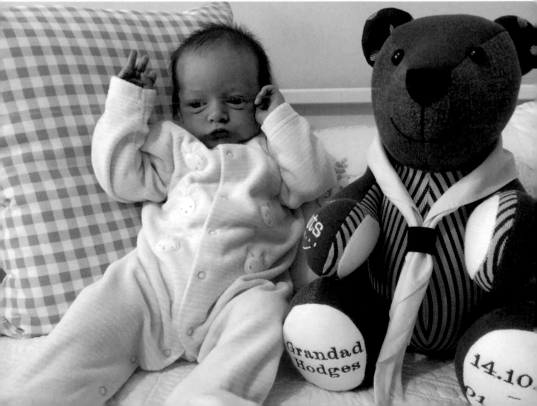

One of our first outings as a family, full of smiles … and a little bit of terror.

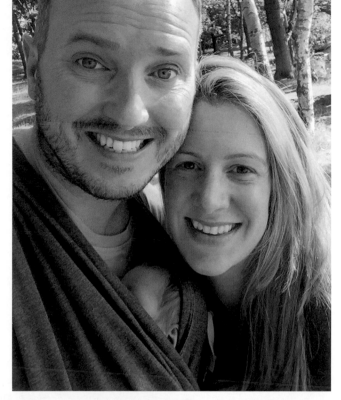

The first Bland family Christmas together, in our festive wear. I hope you and Daddy continue this tradition. Sorry about the outfit!

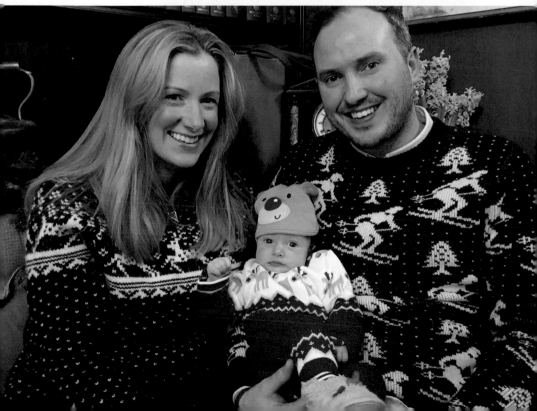

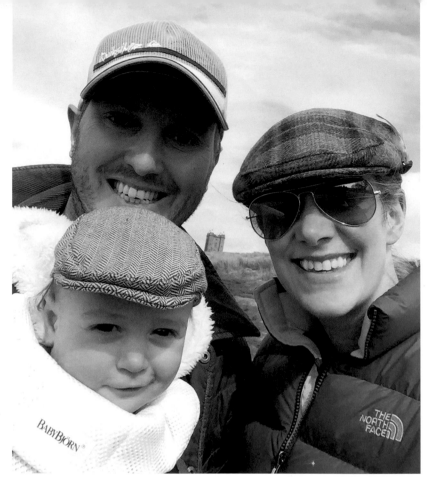

Nothing better than a day out in the countryside. This was us at Lyme Park, resplendent in our matching flat caps.

Your first birthday party – safari-themed for our little adventurer – with the cake that your mummy lovingly made.

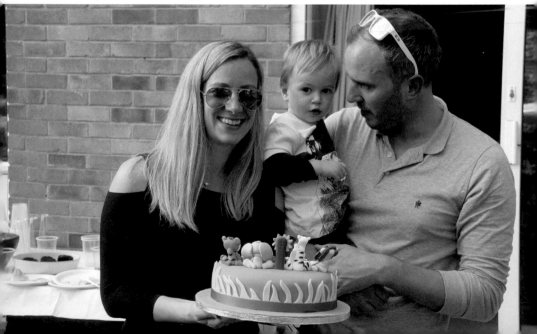

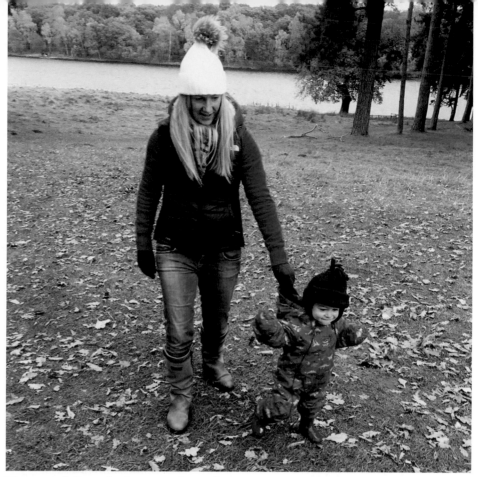

Bittersweet feelings: the day you took your first tentative steps outside, and the last day before I found out I had cancer.

I'm always here to give you a hug, my Freddie.

My two perfect boys.

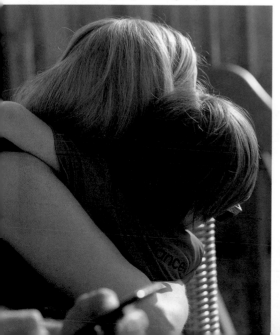

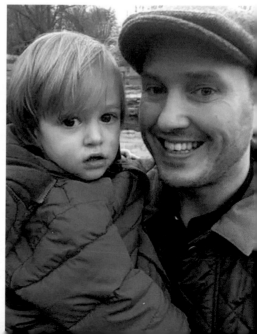

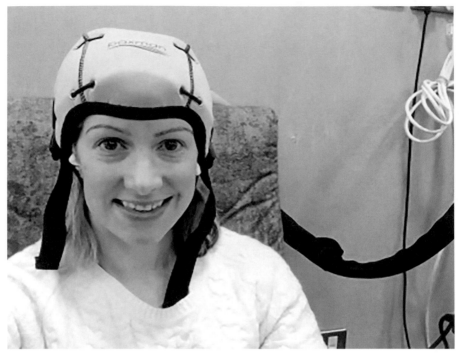

The incredible Paxman cold cap, which helped me to keep so much of my hair.

I didn't feel like a superwoman all the time, but in January 2017 I had just finished my first course of chemo at Macclesfield Hospital and things were looking up.

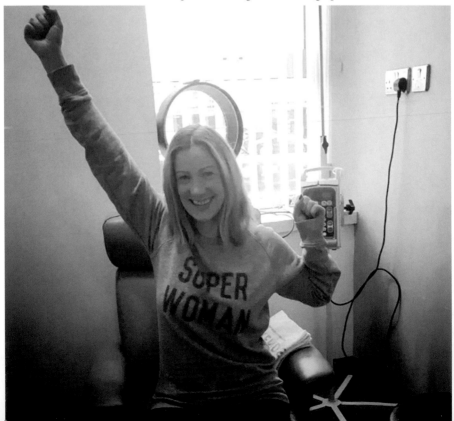

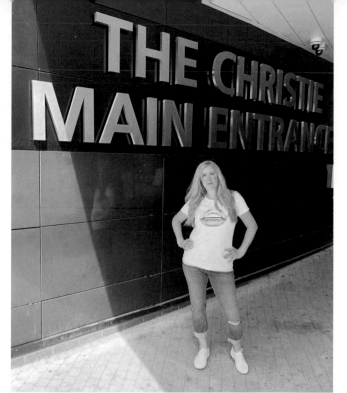

Arriving at the Christie in Manchester, with my game face on and ready to fight.

At the Christie again. This scan would determine whether my trial had been successful. Just one of many scans Mummy had during her treatment.

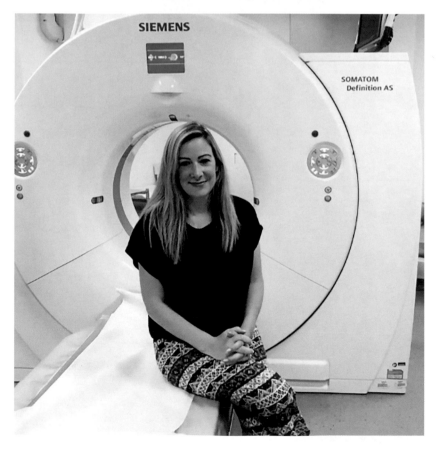

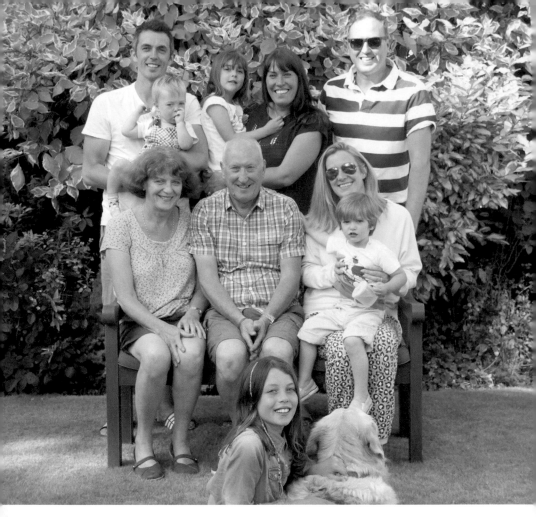

A gorgeous family day with the Bland and Harrison clans.

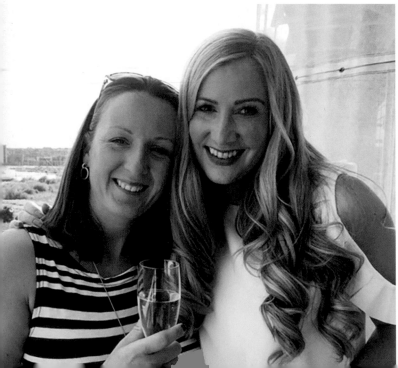

Mummy showing off her new princess hair with one of my Welsh girls, Rachel May, in Cardiff.

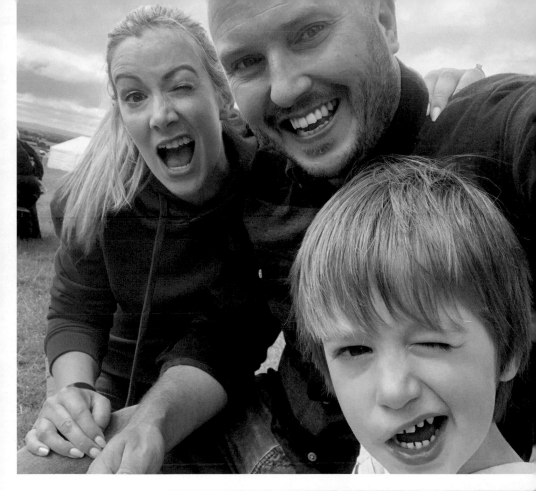

The three best friends that
anyone could have, forever.
There's nothing a little bit of
silliness can't fix, my Fred.

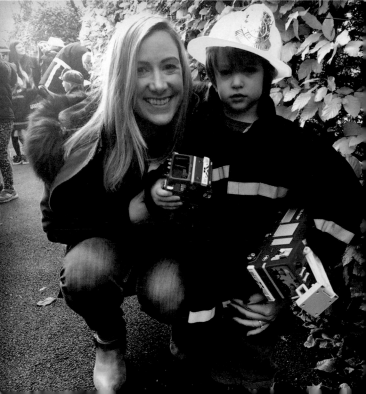

Ready to be a hero, our
very own Fireman Sam.

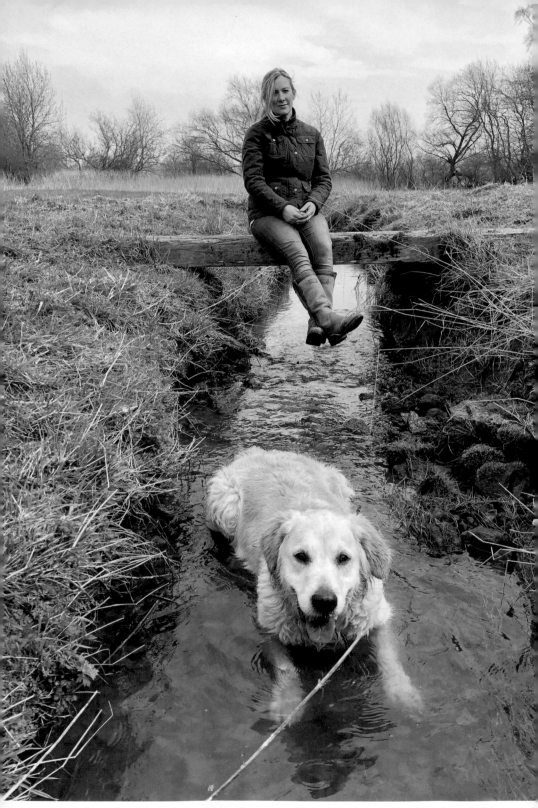

One of your daddy's favourite photos. Country walks with Bodie, what could be better? This one was taken at your Great Uncle Hodges's farm. I loved this bridge.

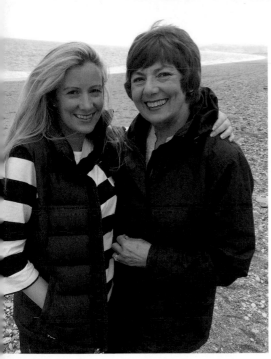

Enjoying a brisk beach walk with your Grandma and chatting away our worries.

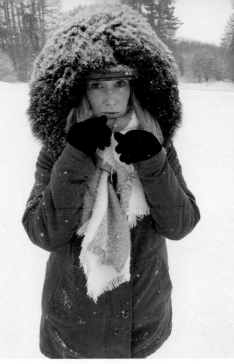

Wrapping up warm on a fortieth birthday trip to the beautiful Gleneagles Hotel, Scotland, in January 2018.

With my Welsh girls, celebrating Tracy's beautiful wedding day.

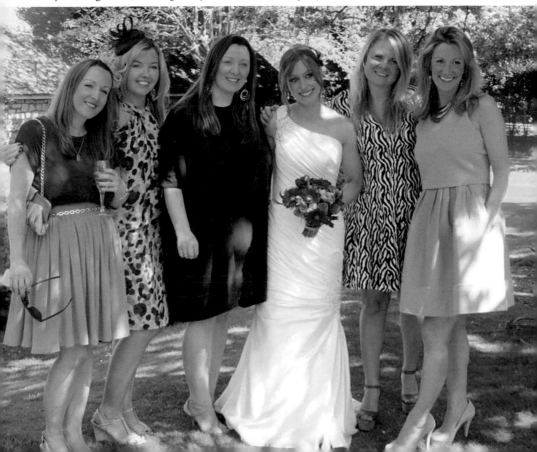

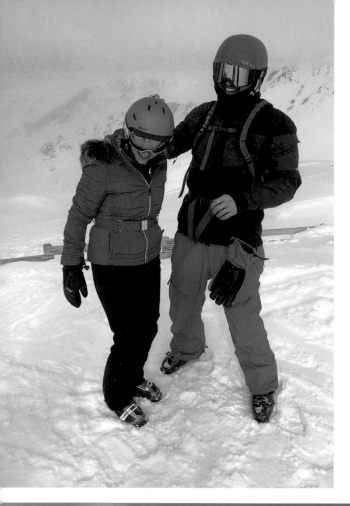

The holiday I didn't think I would be able to make: a ski trip to Méribel with Daddy in January 2018. I couldn't have been happier to hit the slopes.

Enjoying the wilderness and a break from treatment in January 2018.

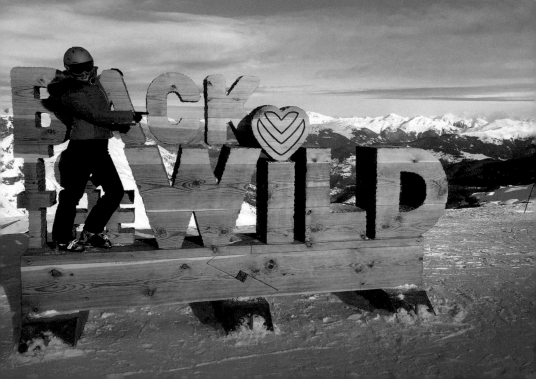

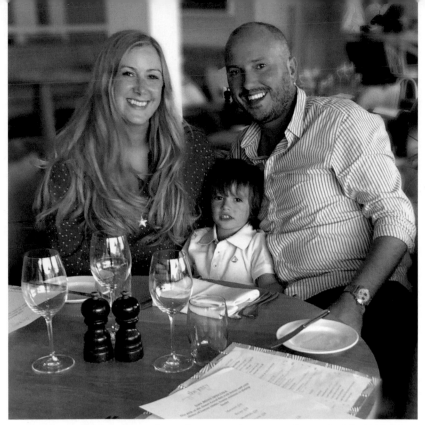

Our last holiday in Salcombe, a place very close to our hearts, in July 2018. I hope you return here with your daddy every summer and have as much fun as we did.

Always taking us on adventures, sea-faring in Salcombe in 2018. You loved to try and drive the boat – but your steering left a bit to be desired!

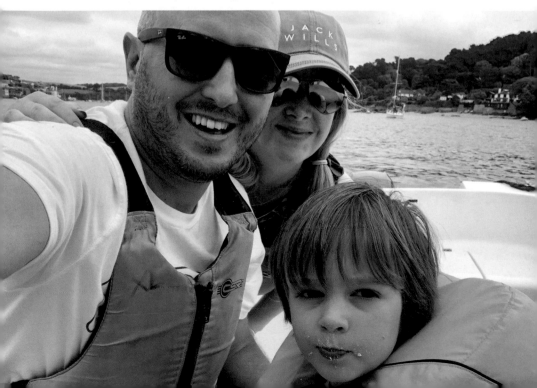

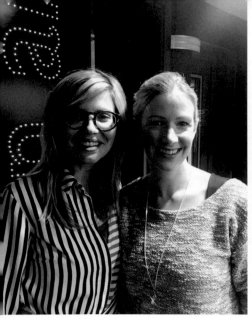

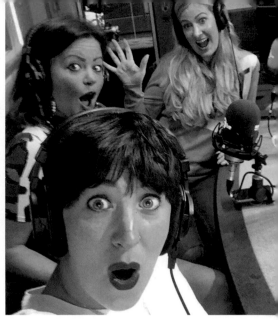

Relaxing after a radio show with Emma Barnett.

One of the first episodes of *You, Me and the Big C* with the glorious Lauren Mahon and Deborah James (aka Lozza and Debs).

We had no idea how successful it would become – we just loved each other's company from the first episode and found comfort in our shared experiences.

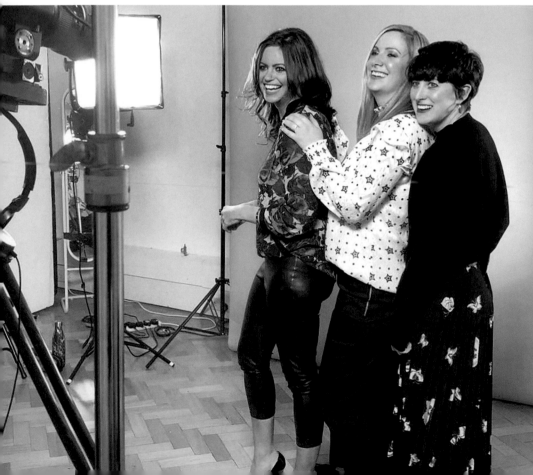

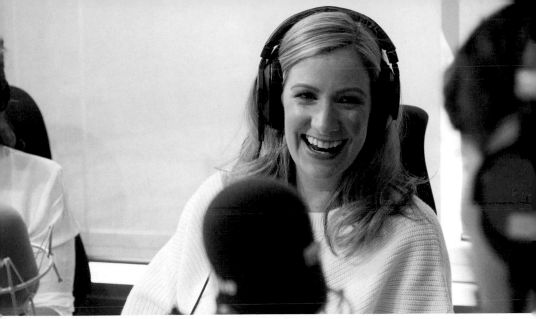

There were days when I didn't feel up to recording, but the support and laughter in the studio always left me rejuvenated.

I am so proud of what we achieved with the podcast, and I hope it continues to inspire people to speak openly and honestly about cancer.

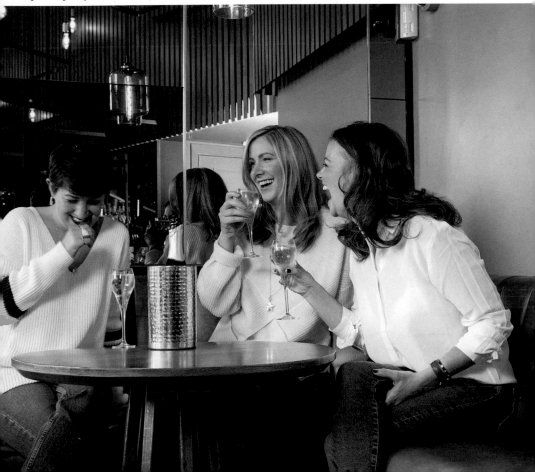

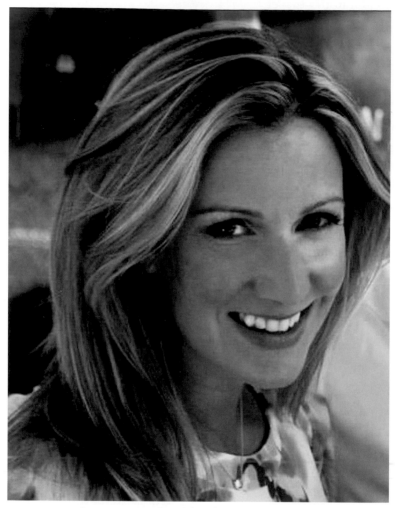

I never expected my life to be cut so short, Fred,
but I ended my forty years with a big smile.

I loved the different modules of my degree where I studied anything from film to newspapers, broadcast journalism and even one on *Star Trek*. I've told you I'm strictly a reality-TV kind of gal and felt I'd been a bit conned into signing up. All the pre-course info had said that students would be studying a major drama series of the twentieth century. Now in my head I'd been thinking along the lines of *Dynasty* … *EastEnders*, maybe. So it was a bit of a shock when the big reveal came during the first lecture and the programme turned out to be *Star Trek*. I raised a tentative hand when the lecturers asked if we had any questions: 'Does it matter if we've never seen an episode of *Star Trek*?' They replied brusquely, 'No, not at all!' – trying to keep the numbers up on the course, I think.! But do you know what? I actually enjoyed the process of analysing different episodes and series, and I finished the module a bit of a fan of Patrick Stewart and *Star Trek: The Next Generation*!

All good things must come to an end and after our three years together in Cardiff it was time to part ways and head for jobs, holidays and further education. I wore my mortar board and gown to pick up my FIRST CLASS HONOURS DEGREE – I shout it here, as once you're in work nobody cares what degree you got. We'd survived, fed ourselves, not got alcohol poisoning (just), done a bit of work and made friends for life.

* * *

I took a year out after uni to go travelling in Australia with Max – this was funded by Grandma and Grandad as a reward for working hard and getting a First (just dropping that in there again!). I'll come back to that trip and the other places I've visited a bit later. We returned tanned and refreshed in the new millennium year. I broke my broadcasting teeth (not literally, luckily) at Bridge FM that I told you about earlier.

And suddenly the summer had rolled around and I started getting messages from the other postgraduate students who would be on my course in Preston. We'd been given a list of phone numbers from the uni and from that we were expected to form into the groups that we would live in over the next year. I ended up with three others: Nadine, Grace and Danny. It was the first time I'd be living with a boy! We found a nice little end-of-terrace and the deal was done. The drive to uni this time took a little longer than the journey to my halls in Cardiff. Mummy was branching out, Fred, bit by bit, stretching my dragon wings and flying that cosy Welsh nest.

We settled into our new home where Danny – a larger-than-life Scouser who used to sell cars – could fill a room with his presence. When cleaning rotas were made he freely admitted that he didn't really do cleaning. So we came up with an ingenious plan: if he promised to clean the toilet every week then he would be absolved from other household cleaning duties. He practically bit our hands off.

It was time to get started on the real work – of learning my trade as a broadcast journalist. I'd chosen the University of Central Lancashire as it had brand-new well-equipped radio and TV studios. It was so much fun – it never felt like work. The North West is a busy, well-populated area with plenty of local radio stations. So off the back of my newsreading work at Bridge FM I managed to get some freelance newsreading shifts in Manchester on Key 103 and Magic, which kept me busy and gave me plenty more experience. I was always told I had a 'great voice for radio' – not to be confused with the slur 'great face for radio'. During that year I was able to develop my newsreading skills and get more work placements to put on my CV.

The year passed by in a flash and before I knew it I was back in a mortar board and gown collecting my postgraduate degree in Broadcast

Journalism. Surely with all my experience in radio now, getting a job would be easy? As always with me it really wasn't. I took a scattergun approach to applying for jobs – basically anything in the BBC. Some of my applications were answered with a polite 'Thanks, but no thanks', while in others I got as far as the interview stage. But remember, my Fred, I told you how I was NOT GOOD at interviews? At the BBC we call them 'boards', but they're the same as a job interview. There's always a panel of three people waiting to grill you on your knowledge of news and their specialism. I've always said, and I promise this is not sour grapes from me because I never got picked, but interviews just throw up people who know how to sell themselves and are confident in that interview process. I've seen plenty of people who do brilliantly at interview stage, but put them on the job and they flounder. Actually doing the job was, for me, the best way of demonstrating that I was good at it, rather than being the bumbling idiot in the interview room, getting flustered and red-faced while trying to think what skills I had that made me great for the job. I applied for so many BBC local radio jobs in so many different parts of the country that it became a full-time job in itself. And it reached the point where I arrived for some interviews not actually convinced I wanted the job.

I think I hit the nadir with my awful performance at an interview for BBC Three Counties in Luton. You know Mummy is a country girl and it was my first visit to Luton, which seemed so urban. The radio station back then was housed on the upper levels of a tower block and I had to buzz to be allowed into the building. I sat waiting to be called for the interview and thought, I really don't want this job. It was lucky then that I could have had a degree in failing interviews at that point, so it wasn't too much of a stretch to barely answer any of the questions.

It was time to go back to the drawing board. One of my best interviews had been at BBC Radio Gloucester, so I called and asked them for some freelance shifts and they were kind enough to oblige. Then more work came up at BBC Hereford and Worcester, and BBC Swindon and Wiltshire. All were within driving distance from Cardiff so I was able to stay at home as I got my career in order. You see sometimes in life, Freddie, if you can't go over something then it might be easier to go round. All roads lead to the same place. One day, I was reading the news on BBC Swindon and Wiltshire and not two minutes after finishing my first bulletin and sitting back down, a man in a smart suit was at my desk, introducing himself as Tony Worgan, the station editor. He really liked my voice and wanted to offer me more work. That initial six-month contract led on to more and eventually I became BBC staff. No shoddy interviews needed, just a bit of persistence and tenacity. So, remember Freddie, if something feels insurmountable, never give up on it. Just look for that other way round.

* * *

Job acquired and the next level of adulting achieved, it was time for me to make my new home in Swindon! Well, actually, not quite yet. Remember me telling you that when Mummy gets an idea in her head she cannot be diverted from it? I am too stubborn. And for some reason I'd decided I didn't want to live in Swindon but would prefer Bristol instead – a thirty-minute drive down the M4. So I took out a six-month let on a nice little flat – the one in which we nearly couldn't get the sofa up the stairs – but because it was in one of the dodgier areas of Bristol, I never really went out or got any benefit from living there. Just lots of extra petrol driving the Roller Skate back and forth to Swindon. So after my six-month lease was up I admitted defeat and skulked off to Swindon with my tail between my legs. It was one of the best moves I ever made. I loved my little flat in the Old Town part of Swindon. I was always so cosy there. I could walk to work, though I never did because I'm a bit lazy and was always running late, and I was able to socialize with my new friends after work without having to worry about the half-hour trip home!

And there were nights out aplenty! The first person I spoke to when I arrived in the station was Uma and I liked her immediately. She is warm and witty, though strong of mind and won't take any crap from anyone, and has probably missed her calling on the stage as a stand-up. After I'd been there a couple of months, Claire joined us on 'attachment' (a process where the BBC will let you change jobs for a while whilekeeping your old job open) from Cornwall, and was a senior broadcast journalist. Her strict outward demeanour – though we all know now she's a pussy cat underneath – and dismissive attitude earned her the nickname 'Scary Claire', though this was only ever said in jest. And rounding off our group was Rae, super-tall with the looks of a model and the brains of Einstein.

We had such a great time that work never really seemed like work. We were a little more blasé in our professionalism then, as this was back in the day when there were still plenty of old hacks around. It seemed acceptable to go to Longs Bar across the road at lunchtime and have a couple of pints of cider before I would co-present the drive-time show and Uma would produce it. Sometimes I think the alcohol gave us a bit of extra energy on air. Just don't tell the boss!

When management were in meetings and Scary Claire was left in charge of us lot, anything could happen. Yes, she was that person who upon spotting a large red button next to her desk asked, 'What does this button do?' then pressed it before anyone could answer. If she'd waited but a moment someone would have told her that the button was the emergency alarm that was connected straight to the police station. There was a lot of shouting out 'NO! NO! NO!' but there was no way to stop the squad car now racing towards the radio station, its occupants thinking we were all in mortal danger. They arrived and took Claire's overenthusiastic button-pushing in good humour. Claire, on the other hand, remains mortified to this day. We could probably have done with the fire brigade instead of the police as Claire had turned an unnatural shade of red in her mortification. Red, as we know from Fireman Sam, Freddie, is the colour of danger! And what an important life lesson we have learnt here, which is to always check what the big red button does BEFORE you push it.

So Claire had form and has also never lived down the time she practically pushed me out of a taxi in her hurry to get home from a night out. I jest about the pushing, but it was one of those rather hilarious nights which finished with everyone being a bit delirious. As I got out of the cab I somehow tripped and ended up laying on my back on the pavement, stranded like some sort of beetle, unable to move because of the tears of laughter streaming down my face. Uma was no great help as she was doubled over on the pavement unable to breathe through her mirth. This was angering Scary Claire who just wanted to get home, so after a couple of tuts and an appraisal of the situation, like a scene from *Bridget Jones's Diary*, she barked at the driver, 'She's fine! Drive on!' Whenever we bring up this story she is adamant that is not how it happened, but that's how me and Umes remember it. So callous! But so funny.

There are almost too many entertaining stories from our days in Swindon to share, but here are just a few of the more memorable ones. 'The night of two curries' is now legendary in the book of Swindon-based stories. Yep, we were those people who started the night with a curry to line our stomachs, went out for drinks, then saw no reason not to have another curry on the way home to soak up the booze! No wonder my weight was up and down through my twenties (mostly up in Swindon!). This is closely followed by the time we ended the night in a strip club on a Monday. I'm not sure why we were all out on such a big night – perhaps we were celebrating our days off being co-ordinated for once – but it turns out that most places in a little town like Swindon close earlier on Mondays, as you don't generally get a bunch of local-radio folk wanting to drink into the wee small hours. We were told by our taxi driver that the only place open until 1 a.m. was the strip club. So off we trotted for another drink there and within ten minutes we had the girls sat down chatting, as we tried to tell them they were better than this and could do more with their lives. Career advice was given, CV tips too and we left feeling we had done our bit for feminism that night! Also worth a special mention is the night out at Po Na Na where the girls realized on looking more closely at the flyers that I bore a passing resemblance to that night's big act, DJ Lolly. So they sat me down in a booth, told me to look like a DJ and then spent the night bringing poor unsuspecting DJ Lolly fans over for a meet-and-greet. Some looked a little sceptical and I really needed to work on my 'impersonating a DJ' schtick, but I'm pretty sure one or two fell for their persuasive spiel … 'Would you like to buy DJ Lolly a drink? She likes vodka and Red Bull. Yes … a pitcher …'

I've probably lost a few adulting points here, but it was a fun and carefree time. But I didn't want to stay in Swindon for ever. I wanted to take the next step up the adulting ladder and that was to move in with Max in London and push my career on to network radio. One of these worked out, the other didn't! I spent much of my time in Swindon chasing up shifts on BBC 5 Live. It had always been my favourite station and this was back in the day when it was really hard to get on air and every shift was fought over. So I kept on sending in demos to the then boss, Moz Dee, whose reaction was always positive but emails ended with a 'We've got nothing at the moment, but stay in touch'. Well stay in touch I did, for FOUR YEARS. Towards the end I would send poor old Moz at least one demo a month. You could never say your mummy was not tenacious, my Fred. Grandma says I was like a little terrier who wouldn't give up. Finally – I think mainly to stop me spamming his inbox – he agreed to give me some overnight newsreading shifts, the holy grail for me back then. This goes to show, Freddie, that if you really want something you just have to keep trying to get it. It may end up with you playing the long game, like I did, or it may happen sooner. But if you want it badly enough, be that terrier and just don't let go of your dreams easily. For hopes and dreams are what get us through life, my darling.

* * *

At twenty-nine, I arrived in London entranced by its busy, smelly streets and historic monuments and buildings all around. Max had agreed to let me stay with him at his sister's flat in Covent Garden 'for a few weeks', but I just thought this would run on. Turns out it was six weeks, and no more, and I was given my marching orders! We'd been together nearly nine years and there was no sign of him making a commitment, so with a heavy heart I decided to move on. You can't keep on waiting and hoping that someone will change themselves for you and it was clear after all that time that marriage and babies weren't on the cards for us. We remain distant friends who catch up with birthday and Christmas WhatsApp messages. So I dropped back down that adulting ladder as I moved into my friend Rachel's flat in Clapham Common and began living the single life of a twenty-something in the big smoke. I loved the area and taking the bus and the Tube to work. Back then it was such a novelty. Now if I go back I just wonder how on earth I would get you around London without losing you on a sweltering hot Tube!

I was back in the clan with my oldest friends from Wales: my bestie Joanna – blonde-haired, loyal and always there for me, a ball of energy and fun who was working her way up to being a very successful business executive; Lucy – already doing well in fashion-buying with an eye for all the beautiful things in life, sweet, funny and fabulous; Rachel – just settling into a brilliant new job in marketing for movies, and now my landlady and confidante. Then further afield but often in London there was Tracy, who lived High Wycombe way, just on the edge of the commuter belt. She's literally one of the sweetest, nicest people you'll ever meet. She's an intensive-care nurse and I always say if I woke up on the ICU to her smiling face, I'd instantly feel better. She also has a great line in filthy jokes. Then Erica, who had moved to make her fortune in Dubai by then, where she was embracing the ex-pat lifestyle like a pro, looking impossibly glamorous while also remaining kind and generous. And finally lovely Laura, who was the first to fly the nest in our early twenties by moving to the USA to work in hospitality and meet her now husband Jeremy. She's remained the most Welsh of all of us, particularly in terms of her accent which is now Cardiff crossed with an American twang and peppered with words like sidewalk and elevator. She's also the one who will still call us all 'ming-stingers' just like in high school! The one big thing we all had in common was our hobbit-like tendency – and no, I'm not talking ugly hairy feet. They must put something in the water in Wales that makes us Welsh women small, as none of us topped five feet four and a half inches and some were significantly smaller. But never underestimate the little people,

Freddie (your growth chart predicts you will be one of the giants!). In the words of the most brilliant playwright William Shakespeare, in *A Midsummer Night's Dream*, my most favourite play of his (it's a rom-com of course!): 'Though she be but little, she is fierce!'

And never underestimate the power of women either, Freddie. I hope in years to come you will both admire and respect them. We are just emerging into what feels like a time of great change for women with the rise of the Me Too movement (calling out men for sexual harassment) and the Equal Pay for Equal Work campaign (drawing out long-lived inconsistencies in the salaries of men and woman doing the same job). Women are fighting back and taking control of their place in a world that has long been dominated by men. While you may think this extra competition could hinder you in life, Freddie, it shouldn't. I hope you always view women as your equals and treat them with the utmost respect. Never measure their achievements by gender. I got very cross with a male friend the other day when he grudgingly admitted that I was very good at reverse parking … for a girl! No, I am just very good at reverse parking for a human. I made it very clear to him I didn't want him repeating the 'okay for a girl' phrase in your presence again. As you can perhaps tell here, Freddie, I have developed my life ideals and ways of living as I've grown up, and am now becoming more and more of a feminist. This is something to bear in mind as you grow up too. Your ideas and opinions on things will change over the years and that's part of life – we live to question the world around us and those questions are in a constant state of flux.

* * *

There were the obligatory nights out in Clapham at Infernos with its sweaty dance floor and sticky carpets. Drinking horrible shots from little plastic glasses that were in no way needed in our state of inebriation. Losing each other in the massive Clapham Grand which was a cut above with its light-up dance floor – a great place to go if you just wanted to dance and sing yourself hoarse with your mates. The weather was always so hot during the London summers – something I've noticed more since my move north! Weekends were spent lazing on a blanket on Clapham Common with a cool drink and some trashy magazines. Well, it was for the other girls. My first summer in London, of course the hottest one, was spent working weekends and trying to get my foot in the door of various radio stations!

When you're a freelancer, Freddie, sometimes you have to make sacrifices. That summer I definitely came down with 'freelance-itis', a condition where you find it impossible to turn down any shifts you are offered in case a) you don't earn enough money that month or b) you turn down a shift only for someone really good to cover it who then goes on to steal all future work away from you! So the majority of Saturdays and Sundays I would trudge away from the girls on Clapham Common, grumbling as I headed down onto the blisteringly hot Tube.

Most of my weekend shifts were at the LBC studios, which were then situated in Hammersmith. I'd get off the Tube in Holland Park, one of London's most affluent areas, as it was quicker to walk than change lines. The journey was always an enlightening one, clearly demonstrating the wealth disparity among the residents of London. The huge neatly kept mansion houses on Holland Park Avenue made it seem like the area was flush with money, then I'd head down towards Hammersmith and the whole outlook changed. Large houses gave way to small flats and high-rise buildings in the distance. The gift shops and high-end womenswear retailers became launderettes, betting shops and takeaways. And this is how I have found most places I've visited in the UK and abroad to be,

Freddie. In the turn of a corner you can go from great wealth to great poverty, but once you crack down the outer layers the people are just the same underneath and should be treated as such.

After a couple of years living with Rach, the time came to move on as she wanted to set up home with her boyfriend (now husband) Pete. So I began flat-hunting with your Auntie Jo and we found a lovely two-bed flat in Wandsworth Common, where we lived for two happy years. Jo's then boyfriend Ben moved in a few weeks later. I still felt I hadn't quite achieved full adulting at this point. I had no mortgage, no commitments and was living in a rented first-floor flat with no garden or outside space! Luckily, the outside-space quota was filled by our local pub, The Hope, which was situated a five-minute walk away with beautiful views across Wandsworth Common. We'd often head there for Sunday lunch only to be found a good five hours later still there with a white-wine spritzer in hand, enjoying the balmy London evenings. Here we'd often meet up with Tina, Janni and Nikki, three of Auntie Jo's work friends, who became some of my closest friends as well. But piece by inexorable piece, our happy gang began to break off into even happier coupledom, buying homes and getting pregnant – 'peak adulting achieved'. I felt like I was the one who was out of step and couldn't keep up. The BBC's move north came at exactly the right time for me and demonstrates, my Fred, why you should never compare yourself to other people in terms of their lives and achievements. You never know what is coming next in life for you, and I too was about to get my adulting wings complete with husband, wedding, dog, mortgage and baby. My bags were packed and ready to head to Cheshire, meet Daddy and buy our first house together. There was a lot of work to be done on it. Especially in the room with nineteen plug sockets …

Chapter 14

THIS OLD HOUSE

I t was the first time buying a house for me. Daddy had bought a few flats in the past, but they were always going to be temporary bachelor pads, not a family keeper. So this was a really important decision. At the time we'd been living in that happy home in Alderley Edge and we loved the village, so that seemed a good starting area. We soon realized that the type of house we currently occupied was only available to us as a rental and definitely NOT to buy. We looked around everything in our price range in Alderley and found that most were much smaller two-bed terraced homes that needed the loft space converting into a third bedroom. This was a level of building work I wasn't really keen on. I wanted to start with an easy decorating job – turns out there's no such thing. We did find a house we liked towards the edge of the village and near the fields where we walked Bodie. We put in an offer that was right at the top of our price range and was duly accepted. Top-level adulting achieved! For a few weeks …

After losing our first baby around this time I suddenly had an epiphany. Funnily enough, I was in church when it happened. There had been a neat seventies four-bed detached house for sale on the

Knutsford estate where Grumpy and Gran lived and also Auntie Claire, Uncle Mark and their children – your cousins-to-be before you came along. We'd spent the whole time, so far, looking for properties with 'character' but it seems that's what everyone wanted, hence you got a lot less space for your money. Some of those little terraces with their small rooms and single living area downstairs were already starting to make me feel a little claustrophobic. As I tried to picture Bodie trotting around in there among the baby paraphernalia that would soon come with your arrival, that claustrophobia began to turn into a little tension and anxiety in my chest! Despite this, when we had first seen the perfectly looked-after home in Knutsford a few weeks earlier, my reaction was 'I'm not living in one of those seventies boxes!' Well, I've always had a bit of trouble making decisions, my Fred – as your Grandad Hodges would say, 'I used to be indecisive but now I'm not so sure'! So in this epiphany moment I realized that I now felt quite the opposite – I really *did* want to live in a seventies box, and very specifically I wanted to live in THAT one, which I had seen in the months before.

This feeling was backed up by the second viewing of the Alderley Edge house when your grandparents came along too. There were negatives I suddenly noticed – it was an end terrace and right next to a railway line. How could I not have spotted this? The kitchen was lovely with a great side room for a muddy Bodie, but you can't buy a house on its dog room alone. None of your grandparents would have dreamed of telling us not to buy it, but we could tell from their demeanours they weren't keen. Another large problem was that the front garden wasn't fully enclosed and opened out onto a footpath. The back garden was enclosed but only had a tiny patio area that wasn't really suitable for dogs – especially one who only likes to go on grass as he's fussy about his wee splashing up his legs while spending a penny! We had visions of Bodie, who has the high-jumping skills of Zebedee from *The Magic Roundabout,* constantly escaping over that fence. Then, when you little future Freddie arrived, having to be on constant watch over you in that open front garden.

No, this was not a good family starter home. Let's go for the seventies box, without much work needing doing, on the estate where our family all lived and in the catchment area for the lovely Bexton Primary School where your cousins go and where Daddy and Auntie Claire went too. Their first teacher still works there and this seemed the perfect environment in which to bring up our son. And that has become even more important to me now, Freddie, as we know I can't be there for many of these pivotal moments in your life. But Daddy, you and I remain the three best friends – remember that, and sing our little song to yourself when you have a big event at school, because my love stays all around you always. I feel so lucky that we have such wonderful family so close by who will be around to support you 100 per cent and be there for all your big moments – cheering you on for all they are worth.

We pulled out of the Alderley sale and excitedly called the agent about the house in Knutsford to put in a bid. I WANTED that house! But of course, sod's law, it had just sold. Someone had seen its potential a little quicker than me. So, we had to start that whole tedious process of viewings again. Then, at the end of our first lot of viewings – none of which were suitable – the estate agent mentioned there was a place that had literally just come on the market on the Bexton estate. Our little ears pricked up … well, this sounded promising! She gave us the name of the road and it was one Daddy knew and was just around the corner from his family. Well, this seemed just too good to be true. Then she tentatively added, 'It needs a bit of work doing', swiftly followed by 'so it's priced to reflect that'. Ah, damn it. There's always something. Undeterred, we rushed straight over for a viewing.

The house didn't have quite as much 'kerb appeal' as others in the street. It was the only one in that row that hadn't been extended and the front drive was full of plants and trees – not really my thing. Still, we headed in to be greeted at the door by the owner. We were given the grand tour of the house, which was decorated in the nineties style we had feared. It was fair to say there was a lot to change. But to be fair, when someone buys Grandma and Grandad Hodges' house they'll be faced with a similar refurbishment job. If you've lived in a house that long there are some repairs that only make sense to you. Grandma is constantly unable to fix things at home as she can remember Grandad doing something clever to them, but not what that was.

Outside, we had a quick conflab, which mostly involved Daddy pulling a pained face and saying, 'We're going to have to buy it, aren't we?' This was due to the lack of houses popping up for sale on the estate and at such a reasonable price and the fact that we knew of other families looking for houses in the same price range.

The next day we offered the asking price and it was accepted. Our seventies box with nineties decor – exactly what I said I hadn't been looking for – was all ours and there was a LOT of work to be done!

* * *

The first big project was getting the lounge in acceptable order. Grandma and Grandad Hodges were coming to visit and Grandad wasn't feeling terribly well by this point. This room, when we moved in, had a rose-pink carpet, swirly flocked wallpaper in shades of white, silver and pink and a dark mahogany-coloured gas fireplace and mantelpiece. There were two corners of the room where, inexplicably, the wallpaper had been painted white. In another unique touch, there was a huge plank of wood above the big window to raise the height of the curtain rail – an ingenious solution to a problem likely caused by curtains that were a touch long. Beyond that was the temporary wall that had been put up to create a dining room off what should have been an L-shaped lounge/dining area. It even had a sliding door to 'keep out the cooking smells'. Beyond it was a tiny dining room in which you could barely swing a cat, which was decorated in a blinding wallpaper with a huge red-flower pattern. I'm afraid to say that the temporary wall was the first thing to be ripped down. We almost felt bad. Almost.

With the ceiling exposed fully, the seventies Artex swirls took on a new intensity. The plasterer was booked to come asap and smooth out those walls, but not before we had taken out the wall lights and discovered some diagonal wiring behind it! As I'm sure your Grumpy will have trained you by now – and you'll have given it a good go with your plastic tools, no doubt – wiring should always run vertically down from an appliance for safety, so you know you can drill or hammer to the right or left of that line. Seeing as we wouldn't be using any of it, Grumpy made it safe by disconnecting the wires. Then it was plastered over, never to be seen again.

With the carpet pulled out, wallpaper gone thanks to some back-breaking work by Gran, and the addition of those lovely smooth walls and ceiling, it was already transformed. Then a whole load of Farrow & Ball paint was thrown at it all, covering up that mahogany fireplace as well. The carpet was delivered and fitted. New curtains and poles delivered from Laura Ashley – now very much in our favour as we got married in her husband's house! – and it was starting to feel cosy. It had that lovely new-home feeling before it gets filled with clutter and too much furniture.

During this time we had been living the hobo life upstairs. A temporary lounge was set up in what is now your room, Freddie – we just borrowed it for a bit! I made the day bed into a sofa, added a few other sticks of cheap Ikea furniture, a lamp and a TV, and you could kind of forget the deep-red walls trying to give you a migraine and settle back for the evening. We slept in the back bedroom with curtains stapled to the rustic wooden curtain-rail mounts. It was always dark in there and was full of our unpacked moving boxes which created a fun assault course on the way to bed each night, but also helpfully covered up the nineteen plug sockets …

Nineteen plug sockets?! Who could possibly need that number in one room? It had been painted in a very sugary shade of lavender – much like Parma violets. Perhaps they wanted to cover some of it with plug sockets? Now most people don't see plug sockets as a feature, but here they were raised to above the height of the bedside tables, which, to be fair, is kind of a good idea as they can be a right bugger to get to when switching off the night light. Perhaps even more bizarrely, in addition to the many sockets positioned at varying heights across the walls, there were also two blocks of cheap plastic plug sockets in the room. There was a TV set, a DVD player and I presume a VHS player, but that still doesn't explain the other five sockets being needed. It will remain one of life's great unsolved mysteries to me, my Fred.

* * *

Room by room, we stripped off the layers of paper, new carpet and floors were fitted and Farrow & Ball was painted on. Pictures were hung and, bit by bit, it started to feel like our home. Every time we found a wire painted into place – they genuinely were everywhere like a giant spider's web – we'd just start pulling until we got to the end of it and removed it. It was a bit like pulling up ivy. But we were stuck with what would have been the most expensive room to update in the house – the kitchen. And we are still stuck with it now, five years on! It had white cupboard doors in a very nineties style with a white paint outer layer which, after the replacing of a few very sticky baby safety clasps, is now peeling off in a number of spots. The doors all had the cheapest plastic round handles available. In an ingenious bit of engineering two drawers wouldn't open properly as the handles blocked each other. The flooring is your finest grey tile-effect lino. Worktops are the most basic grey Formica. There are the slightly wonky white tiles with a twist-effect top. And what colour to paint the wallpaper liner above this? Why a cherry red, of course! What else? I have always refused to do anything to update the kitchen as it seemed a waste if we were going to do it properly one day. Though I did begrudgingly spend a day repainting that cherry red with a light grey. My eyes just couldn't take the red! Oh and there's the cooker I talked about earlier, which I battle with every year when making your birthday cake. It's become some sort of personal challenge for me to create a moist cake with it. Your next birthday is in a month and I think I may start practising now. Challenge is on, oven of hell. I'd like to see even the great Mary Berry create a moist cake in that furnace.

The bathrooms were the other bits we couldn't afford to update after blowing the wedding budget. The downstairs one is particularly special as the tap only runs cold water and the basin is so small it's impossible to wash even your tiny hands in it, Freddie, without most of the water ending up on the floor!

We'd planned to do all the expensive bits, like those bathrooms, kitchen and an extension, with the next couple of remortgages, but then cancer came along and ruined that party. It means that maybe you will get to help Daddy choose how these rooms will look. The one room I'd like to redecorate before I die is your little room, Freddie. I think it's time for the twee baby owl pictures and stickers to come down and the baby teddies and books to be put away, and something more befitting a three-year-old boy with a love for trucks, tractors and rockets put up in their place. My parting gift to you for the next few years.

We have been so happy in this house, Freddie. Sometimes the kitchen and the bathrooms and the fancy furniture just aren't important. I know Mummy has admitted to liking the finer things in life, but I know in my heart they don't matter. What matters is you, Daddy, me and Bodie. Partners in crime and, between the four of us, wrecking all that lovely expensive paint and furniture, but also having fun together in a house filled with our love for each other. I hope you stay in this house for as long as possible – it was the happy home that love built. But no matter where you move through life, a big piece of me will follow. In my style, in my things and in my love.

Chapter 15

MUSIC, SWEET MUSIC

As you'll have gathered from my many mentions of it in the book so far, Freddie, music has played a huge part in my life and I love it. Nothing can compare to that feeling when a piece of music really touches you and makes your spine tingle. It all started back on those holiday car journeys to Devon and Cornwall and us singing along to Grandad's cassette tapes in the car. It meant I knew most of the words to the Beatles' songs before those of Kylie Minogue's 'I Should Be So Lucky', and the Monkees' 'Daydream Believer' was a classic in my head long before they started playing it as an end-of-night tune at the student union.

I guess you could say my musical 'coming of age' was just as we popped into that cheesy Stock, Aitken and Waterman phase of Kylie, Jason Donovan, Sinitta, Sonia and the like. Not quite what you'd call a 'classic era' of music. I was aware of the New Romantics and synth-pop bands, but only through the stickers in my *Smash Hits* album featuring Boy George, Duran Duran, Spandau Ballet and Adam and the Ants. Though luckily, this mid-to-late eighties entry into music swept me into the path of the Queen of Pop, Madonna, in her classic 'Like a

Virgin' era. I had all her albums on cassette from *Like a Virgin* and *True Blue* to *Like a Prayer*. I had the sparkly, lace fingerless gloves and there's a Polaroid picture of me in Madonna fancy dress in the garden (another of Grandma's creations), with blue sprayed hair and a cut-up sparkly dress, thinking I *was* the Queen of Pop in that moment. I also had a VHS cassette of one of her live tours, from which I would religiously try and copy her dance moves. My attempts were, as I'm sure you'll understand, pretty poor.

Back in the red Sierra with the touring caravan on the back, we had to drive so slowly that Grandad Hodges had plenty of time to introduce us to his favourite music. And at least once every journey we would listen to *Jeff Wayne's Musical Version of The War of the Worlds* – a prog-rock album, which was released in the year I was born. A retelling of the story in H. G. Wells's sci-fi classic, *The War of the Worlds*, in which Martians visit earth and try to take it over, it features the spoken voices and vocals of Richard Burton, David Essex and Justin Hayward, among others. It both terrified and thrilled me in equal measure. And I remember sitting in the car listening to much of it with my hands over my ears. Those opening couple of bars of 'The Eve of the War' will always give me goosebumps and a sense of foreboding – the repetitive cries from the Martians of 'ULLA!!' would terrify my six-year-old self. But then interspersed with that were wonderful heart-wrenching songs like 'Forever Autumn', which I think reminded Grandma and Grandad of losing Uncle Bobby, and we'd all sing along to it with a tear in our eye.

Once we'd all worked ourselves up into a terrified frenzy with *The War of the Worlds*, we'd take things down to a smoother, cheerier level with perhaps a bit of the Everly Brothers – who could resist a bit of Don and Phil? Grandad seemed to be drawn to acts with a bit of a country vibe – I suspect it was all the guitar playing. And they wrote some beautiful songs like 'All I Have To Do Is Dream', 'Wake Up Little Susie' and our family favourite 'Let It Be Me', which always makes me tear up. You see, Freddie, there's a lot of power in music. It can be very emotive and can take you immediately back to times and places where those songs meant something to you. I hope you recall the love that passed between all three of us like an electric current as we cuddled up tightly before bedtime and sung 'Three Best Friends'. Or those moments where I sang the 'Bland family sleeping song' to you to help you to get back to sleep, and the moment I'd stop singing your head would pop straight up asking for the BoBo song again. It started with your amazing Gran and Grumpy singing it to Daddy and Auntie Claire, then we've all sung it to you little ones in slightly different versions. Ours goes slowly and repetitively (in the hopes of boring you off to sleep) …

> Bobo Freddie …
> Bobo Freddie …
> Bobo Freddie …
> Mummy's little boy.

Then sometimes I'd freestyle a second verse:

> Sleepy time, Freddie …
> Sleepy time, Freddie …
> Sleepy time, Freddie …
> I'd like to go downstairs.

This would be sung ad infinitum until you nodded off! To be fair it was no Everly Brothers song in either tune, styling or skill, but you liked it and you sometimes try and sing it yourself now to your little pal Annabelle, who we went on holiday with recently, and it is one of the cutest things ever!

The Everlys played a number of times in the St David's Hall in Cardiff, so I ended up seeing them live three times! I'm not sure that's something to boast about while in your teens, but I didn't care. They may not have been top of the cool list, along with going to a gig with your parents, but I loved hearing them sing live and their harmonies and guitar-playing were just too good to be missed. Later, as I went through my twenties and thirties, Grandad became a massive Status Quo fan – he was always about the guitars – and as they seemed to tour in December and his birthday was mid-October, a couple of tickets always made a top gift.

Through my teenage years at school I'd say I lost my way musically a little. I thought I was being cool listening to a lot of dance music, but in hindsight I wish I'd been expanding my musical tastes by going to more live gigs. I think this was a sign of me being a bit shy and a bit of a follower back then. I genuinely wasn't a huge fan of the repetitive beats of most dance music, but loved anything with a good vocal. A good example was RuPaul's 'House of Love', which one of Uncle Matthew's friends had on a picture disc – I knew every word. This was the era where record decks were the thing for any dance fans and the world and his wife wanted to be a DJ! But I feel I missed out on a lot of the teenage angst music like Nirvana and later Oasis, who I came to as something of a latecomer but now love their utterly anthemic tracks. And of course because I'm now an honorary northerner! My personal favourite – away from all the obvious big tracks – is 'She's Electric'. Always a volume up, 'sing at the top of my voice' track.

* * *

In my late twenties, after I moved to London and had any number of gigs at my fingertips, I began to listen to more indie pop-rock acts like

Paolo Nutini, who I saw at the Brixton Academy. I also got into the early Arctic Monkeys. 'I Bet You Look Good on the Dancefloor' is still guaranteed to get me dancing – got to prove the Monkeys right, eh? My other favourite track from that first album is 'Mardy Bum'. You'll recognize that grumpy partner in the song – she sounds a bit like you and me, Fred. Stuck in our little moods!

Then, of course, how could we go any further without mention of my favourite band of all time, the Killers. It's hard to know when I first began liking their music. They suddenly slotted into my life as my number-one band where every gig was like a religious experience to me. I may not believe in a god any more, but I do believe in the divine power of music and most of their gigs (I've seen them a good nine times now) are spent with my hands held aloft and punching the air in their direction, mesmerized by the feeling. And this, Freddie, is the wonderful power that music can have over you and why I'd love you to listen to as much as possible and find your niche or a broad genre of songs that make you feel something. Whether it be happy, sad or in love, music can be such a life-enriching experience – the soundtrack to everything you do.

I started seeing the Killers when they were on tour after the release of their second album, *Sam's Town*, and watched Brandon Flowers – the lead singer – grow from the man who some music journos thought was too quiet and not charismatic enough to be a frontman. He was all about the sparkly feathered jackets in those days, as if trying to earn his place there. The band hails from Las Vegas, Nevada, a fact that always works its way into every gig and a place where I've always wanted to see them play. And through the next couple of albums *Day & Age*, *Battle Born* and now *Wonderful Wonderful*, Flowers owns the stage with power, grace and swagger. His voice is incredible, such a perfect tone live, and his strut around the stage during 'The Man', in a gold suit and glasses reminiscent of Elvis, is quite astonishing. Ronnie Vannucci Jr is like Animal from the Muppets on drums – pretty sensational live.

My love for the Killers has also managed to rub off on Daddy – he has fallen for their music hook, line and sinker and it feels wonderful (or should that be 'Wonderful Wonderful'!) to give someone else the joy of their music. I hope one day they'll still be touring and Daddy can take you along. Let me give you this image … I would frequently be standing (definitely if it was a festival and not hygienic to sit on the grass!) singing all their songs right back at the band, at the top of my voice, hands in the air with a lot of pointing and looking euphoric. As I've said, I am no longer religious after all that has happened, but this was my church and this was where I came to sing and to feel. I hope you get that same experience from seeing them if you can one day.

Recently I appeared on the Radio 2 breakfast show, *Good Morning Sunday*, with the Reverend Kate Bottley and Jason Mohammad to talk about how I was coping with my terminal diagnosis and what was getting me through. As part of this I was allowed to choose a song to play – a real accolade to be able to take over the coveted BBC Radio 2 playlist. Of course it had to be a Killers track and then I happened upon the perfect one which will forever be my favourite Killers song from here on out. It's called 'A Dustland Fairytale' and is all about Flowers's mother and father – how they met, fell in love and he became a devoutly religious man when 'revelation set his soul on fire'. His mum in later years became very ill with brain cancer and in the song Brandon is begging her not to go yet. This is one to look up on Google, Freddie, and I hope you love it as much as I do.

It just seemed to fit in so well with what I hope this book will give you. Details. If you should ever want to write a song about your mummy and daddy, and how they met and fell in love, then you have all the information that you need here now. Or it may be a poem or a book or a work of fiction. Any creative process. I hope I am leaving behind for you some of my legacy here, my Freddie, so you don't feel you've ever forgotten it or didn't know how our life was.

I've met Brandon just the once when he came to do an interview on BBC 5 Live in Salford and your friend Auntie Dawn (of the cute elf outfit mentioned earlier) helped me to track him down and introduce us. He was an utterly charming and lovely man who looked only slightly taken aback at my fan-crazed ramblings! I was about six months' pregnant with you at the time and had just come off a breakfast shift reading the TV bulletins for BBC North West Today, so was a little delirious from the 3 a.m. start. I explained to him that I'd been playing Killers music into my womb using my iPhone in the hope of making you an instant mini-Killers fan when you came out. Brandon managed to hide his surprise well with just a slight eye raise and a 'WOW!' and obliged me by taking a couple of snaps with his stalker, which are still among my most treasured photos. And then he was dragged off by his team to his next commitment, leaving me in his perfectly featured, wonderfully coiffured hair and fabulously smelling wake. So you've kind of met him too, Fred, albeit from inside Mummy's tummy!

I sadly missed the last Killers gig I had booked – a big stadium one in Bolton of all places – but to be honest it might have been a bit emotional for me, feeling that it might be the last time I ever saw them. It wouldn't do to be weeping through 'All These Things That I've Done' rather than shouting at the top of my lungs. Seeing that I was in hospital at the time, for breathing problems with said lungs, it really wouldn't have felt quite right.

I think the highlight of my times seeing the Killers was watching them headline the Isle of Wight Festival in 2013. There is nothing that quite compares to seeing your favourite band headline the Saturday night of a festival. There's an immersive quality to standing in the dark in a field among thousands of other like-minded people and I was determined to take in every moment of the experience. I sang myself hoarse, held my arms in the air until my shoulders ached and absorbed every savoured second. When the band were finished Uncle James, always one for a wry comment, turned to me – eyebrows raised – and said, 'I knew you liked the Killers, but you REALLY like the Killers!' My only response was a nod – yep, I REALLY love the Killers.

I also really love a good festival. We had started going to the Isle of Wight Festival a few years before, when Auntie Jo and Tina were able to get free tickets through a friend. A free ticket saves you vast amounts of money as they're pretty expensive. Then I managed to get on a VIP list through a press contact, so always had a pair of VIP wristbands each year. The best thing about these was it meant we had access to a nice bar with sofas outside it and the all-important flushing toilets with soap and hand towels that were cleaned on a regular basis. I think I did four years or so at the Isle of Wight without having to use a Portaloo, save for a quick stop on the walk back from the stage to the campsite if desperate, and it was an experience not to be repeated! I can still feel the germs and smell the horrific smell.

Each year we learnt more about getting the best camping spot, after arriving late one time and being stuck right at the back of the main campsite, which added at least an hour to the walk back from the main stage. The next year we booked into Tangerine Fields where they pitch your tents for you in neat rows with inflatable mattresses and have flush-toilet blocks, warm shower blocks and even a hair pamper station with hairdryers and straighteners – luxury! Unfortunately that was the year it chucked it down with rain, so it meant all of these little luxuries had to be unplugged as the rain rendered them a danger to our frizzy locks. We'd also stupidly just booked a row of small two-man tents, which made getting in and out with muddy wellies a tricky and back-breaking operation. It was so muddy that year that it took twice as long to get anywhere through the boggy mud and James I think regretted his choice of a demi-welly – perfect for dog walking in London, but not so good for deep festival mud as it oozed in over the top. The following year we nailed it with a six-man tent at the Tangerine Fields, which meant we each got a little bedroom with a living area in the middle that you could actually stand up in! We could sit in our camping chairs in comfort even if there were a few spots of rain. Of course there weren't any that year – whenever you're fully prepared for rain, the sun beams down! But we weren't complaining. The sun shining on you at a festival is like nothing on this earth. We had such a fun weekend that year.

The Isle of Wight Festival isn't everyone's cup of tea, but I think it's where we fitted in. I've never done Glastonbury but it looks too big and a bit too hippy for my tastes. I think I'd spend the whole weekend just searching for my tent in those massive fields! V Festival is perhaps the opposite end of the scale and is 'peak Towie' – not my scene at all! So the Isle of Wight sits somewhere in the middle of the two. We've seen some great current bands there like Bastille, Foo Fighters and some old rockers like Tom Petty and the Heartbreakers and Bon Jovi – screaming 'Living on a Prayer' at the top of your lungs in a dark field with a bunch of strangers is always a moment you won't forget! It's good to have fun with your music, Freddie, and let it take you to different places, meet new people and have new experiences.

* * *

On the other end of the spectrum, you'll know I've mentioned your dad's and my love of cheesy music and that, of course, has to extend to a musical or two. I've never been one of these artsy types who wants to see a play on Broadway or in the West End. Give me a musical any time of the week. Our favourite is *Les Misérables*, of course – the king of the musical genre. Every song is so catchy and makes you want to sing along, while the story has such passion and the staging is always a wonder! Your dad loves the film version with its live-action singing, though I am less of a fan as I prefer the more pure sound of a true stage voice.

We're oft to be found singing in the car to the show tunes. I've also been a huge fan over the years of *The Phantom of the Opera* – I used to love to play 'The Music of the Night' on the piano. I'm also in love with 'Defying Gravity' from the musical *Wicked* and when home alone – your presence excepted – I'll try and give it the full, belting, top-of-the-range sing-along and pretend I am Idina Menzel. Obviously, to your ears listening in it would sound more akin to Florence Foster Jenkins unfortunately. If there is one thing in life that I have always wished I could do, Freddie, that is to sing. I mean really sing with tone and power and in tune! I sound okay and can vaguely hold a tune, but not with any great range or power. The beauty in my voice only seems to come out in the spoken word, hence becoming a newsreader! But I've always thought what a wonderful feeling it must be to be able to sing like a pro – how your heart must soar with every note you hit.

I hope your life is still filled with the sound of music, my Freddie. I hope you and Daddy continue to listen to the songs I love. And I hope you find your own new songs that will fill your heart with joy and love. Because when, in life, things seem to be going wrong, the right song can come along and make everything feel just that little bit better again. Maybe those songs will be sent by me from out there in the ether somewhere. That's the power of music, it transcends barriers and it's a nice little thought to have, isn't it my darling, that Mummy could be sending little musical messages to you from somewhere in the big out there?

Chapter 16

THE WORLD IS YOUR OYSTER

The best way to find and connect with Mummy in the big out there, my Fred, is to get out there and explore it. Having led a fairly sheltered upbringing travel-wise, what with Grandma's fear of flying, I was chomping at the bit to see some more of the incredible world we are blessed to live in. And so I took every opportunity that funds would allow, especially after the typical cheap and boozy holidays in Magaluf, followed by another in Rhodes.

Next up was a somewhat longer and more cultured tour – well, full of Aussie culture – when I travelled for four months in Australia. My gift from your grandparents for getting my degree and attaining First Class Honours (got to mention it here repeatedly as, remember, no one ever cares again!) was the funding to go travelling in Australia. So Max and I set off on what seemed like an incredible, exotic path, having never been further than Europe before. To break up the massively long flight we stopped off in Singapore for a couple of nights. What a blaze of noise and lights that was – a real zinger on the senses. Max wanted to buy a posh camera lens, so a lot of the time was spent trudging around numerous electrical goods' malls looking for the right thing and trying not to get ripped off. We'd heard tales of people taking home the boxes containing what they thought were the correct item only to get there and find a cheaper and inferior product inside. It was a minefield! The rest of the time was spent seeking out delicious Asian food and making the most of a luxury hotel before beds and rooms became a little more basic!

Before we knew it we were on another plane journey and headed for our big experience in the land down under. We were starting in Cairns and had booked into a nice little hostel on the edge of town where were we able to have our own room – result! Every night we'd head down to the Woolshed bar near the Cairns Marina with our free dinner ticket from the hostel and would have a pretty great bowl of food. I just had to Google the name of it and discovered it is celebrating its twenty-fifth anniversary in 2019. I was there in 1999, so it was just a few years old when I arrived. After dinner we were introduced for the first time to the delights of Aussie beers and measures by the group from our hostel. Beer was bought in pitchers and poured into 'pots', which are small plastic cups or schooners, slightly larger than and something akin to a half-pint pot. Either way, if it was VB (Victoria Bitter) you were drinking out of them you'd end up with a banging headache the next morning. We soon learnt to switch to Tooheys which had far fewer impurities.

Now I should point out that this first night out was off the back of two flights, and after arriving at 5 a.m. Australian time my body clock didn't know if it was coming or going. But after a few pitchers of beer at the Woolshed and a lot of dancing to the same songs we would come to hear over, and over, and over, and over, in all Aussie bars nationwide I gave myself up to the table top, dancing to the Proclaimers' 'I'm Gonna Be (500 Miles)', 'My Sharona' by the Knack, and 'Down Under' by Men at Work. We finally stumbled back to our hostel at God knows what hour and woke with banging hangovers (we obvs didn't change from the VB – idiots), which were now combined with a serious case of jet lag, a state that took a good week to get over. A sage bit of advice, Freddie – avoid the strong alcohol when you arrive somewhere with jet lag. Get yourself back on local time and you'll be good to enjoy your first few days much more than we did! We dragged ourselves around the tourist attractions near Cairns, which is in itself not much to write home about, and we fed the obligatory kangaroos at the safari park. One of the most impressive things about Australia is how different its animals are to ours. Kangaroos, koalas, cassowaries, wombats and crocodiles are not like anything you'd bump into on Wandsworth Common while out walking the dog!

A few days in, we'd recovered enough to start training for one of the main activities we'd come to this area for – deep-sea diving. All the basic training took place in a pool and classroom under the teaching of a rather cool dude called Grant. He got us through all the basics, including how to read the fiendishly complicated dive tables which tell you how much air you've used and how much is left. We practised taking our masks off in the pool and taking out the regulator (the round bit at the end of a tube you breathe through) – 'The Reg' in Grant speak – and putting it back in again. Then we were off for three nights on our liveaboard yacht. All was pretty cosy and swanky inside and I was happy and excited to be heading out to sea! Max, on the other hand, was turning a vulgar shade of green that I had not seen on a human face before and was leaning over the back of the boat being very, very sick.

Travel sickness is not something I've ever suffered from, Freddie, and I hope you've taken after your mummy in this regard because poor

Daddy will get queasy at the tilt of a high-speed Pendolino train – the clue is in the 'leano' bit. It's a lot easier to be able to read in a car and look at the beautiful horizon from a boat without leaning down to be sick every five minutes! The yacht started slowing down sometime around 9 a.m., which meant we had arrived at our first dive stop. Still decidedly green, Max enquired of Grant as to whether it a wise decision for him to carry out. 'Ah naah mate, it's fine. You can vom through y'reg,' came the broad Aussie reply. And so we went through the ungainly process of hauling ourselves into our wetsuits and shrugging on our buoyancy aids and oxygen cylinders, and before we knew it we were being shoved into the water and surrounding reef on our first qualifying deep-sea dive!

I was most awe-inspired by what I could see fifteen metres down under the surface of the Great Barrier Reef and also a little bit terrified. We'd had our little books out ready to identify all the different types of colourful fish we might encounter. The clownfish and butterflyfish that we saw have since been made famous in the animated film *Finding Nemo*. As we approached the sea anemones the clownfish first would aggressively shoot out defending their families. We'd often see the ungainly features on the ancient faces of the moray eels roaring out at us too. But my favourite moments were those when we nipped off with Grant into more open waters and found the turtles, who were so graceful cutting through the water and who, it seemed, were pulling us along in their wake. This also threw us into the path of the deep ocean shelf as the shallower reef dropped off into the darkness of the depths – exciting and terrifying as the water got blacker and blacker. From here would emerge the reef sharks, mainly blacktips, and my breathing rate and use of oxygen would suddenly whoosh straight up.

I was so in love with challenging my fears with diving. This is something I told you I've always done, Freddie, and something I would like you to do when things scare you a little. Face your fears head on and the feeling of achievement you get when you win your own mental battle is just the most amazing one.

So we continued down the standard east coast backpacker trail until we reached the Whitsundays, a beautiful collection of seventy-four continental islands off the Queensland coast about 560 miles north of Brisbane. The prime backpacker trade from here, based out of Airlie Beach, is liveaboard sailing trips, and after being bitten by the diving liveaboard bug we decided that would be our main priority here – three days on another liveaboard yacht and just a day out on a sailing ship, but before that something else caught my eye …

The one thing I had said I would NOT do when we arrived in Australia was a skydive. Everything else I was up for, but that seemed a little too far out of my comfort zone. But that first morning of our stay in the Whitsundays, the skies were bright and blue and clear. The weather was set for it and a little idea started working its way into my head that if I was ever going to try sky-diving then this was the moment, under bright blue skies looking over the beautiful, white, squeaky silica sand of the Whitsundays. So I made a call home to Grandma to get her thoughts – ridiculous idea, I know, but she said if I could guarantee it would be 100 per cent safe then to go for it while I was there. She must have been having some sort of out-of-body experience back in Wales because obviously there was no way I could promise 100 per cent safety on a skydive, but I did and we carried on with our little charade. If she'd seen me about an hour later, tandem-strapped to a hairy fella who I'm pretty sure was stoned in the back of a rickety plane, then she may have changed her mind! At one point I thought it prudent to give my tandem driver a little nudge on the shoulder, just to check he was awake and compos mentis for his important job of gliding me softly to the ground behind him, and the grunt he gave showed me he was. Next thing I knew I was hanging feet first out of the side door of the plane as old stony manoeuvred us into free fall. My breath was immediately whipped out of my lungs and my head whiplashed back as we dropped at the speed of a stone and a stoner.

I had the unfortunate experience of watching Max jump first, as he had the camera attached to his tandem diver, and to see him plummet at top speed away from the plane gave me a real sense of how fast free fall was going to be. And that was supersonic! So just as I was getting my breath back, it was time to pull the cord on the parachute to put the brakes on. And it seemed that there were just those extra couple of seconds where I felt like bellowing 'PULL THE CORD! PULL THE CORD!' But this highly trained professional did it at just the right moment and we were briefly wrenched back up into the air before beginning our graceful swooping loops down, gazing at the beautiful Whitsunday Islands below. The feeling of elation to have made it down (almost) in one piece was brilliant. Just that one bump down in the field – legs up to avoid breaking them (always a wise peice of advice) – and I was down safely. I couldn't stand up for my legs shaking as I fought to get the air back in my lungs, but I had done it! Another mental thrill-seeking challenge I thought I'd never do ticked off the list.

This comes back to the thread I've been weaving throughout this book for you, Freddie, my sweetheart. The challenges you take on in life don't have to be the big show-off moments that you film on the way down. Some of them will seem insignificant to other people, but you will know when you've challenged your body or your mind and won. Keep piling up those little achievements, rock by rock, and soon you will have a wall of armour that can protect you through the rest of your life.

So our trip up and down the east coast of Australia continued. Should you ever want to follow it one day it's the well-worn backpacker route of Cairns, up to a beautiful rainforest area called Cape Tribulation (really off the beaten track), Townsville and Magnetic Island, and Airlie Beach with its skydive, three-day dive liveaboard and a day out on a huge sail boat. Then we went down, through and past Brisbane, stayed in the 'Vegas of the Gold Coast', Surfers Paradise, a few days longer than we planned but we found a nice hostel and some fun friends so were flexible! Then we finished at the far more hippy and beautiful hangout of Byron Bay.

We nipped over from Brisbane to Melbourne on a quick (four-hour) flight – nowhere is close in Australia! I'd been told I'd love Melbourne, but actually someone broke into our hostel one morning while we were having breakfast and stole our camera bag – luckily, that was all, and the expensive lenses and passports got left behind as I think we disturbed them. But I never felt safe there after that and I couldn't let go of the fact that all the video footage of our trip – some of it quite hilarious, I might add – was gone. Then there was a week in Sydney admiring the Harbour Bridge and the Opera House, which are pretty darned impressive! I have been back on a brief trip since to visit the west coast of Australia too. Perth I found nothing to write home about like many big cities, but the wine tour area to its south is worth a visit.

* * *

One city I can recommend, and have always wanted to visit in warmer climes, is New York! I headed to the Big Apple in February 2004 with Auntie Jo, Lucy and Rach, after spending eight days in the slightly warmer Deep South environs of Hilton Head Island. I'll come back to my New York trip later, but first I must tell you about when our little gang of four Welsh girls went on our first big holiday adventure, Fred, to South Carolina! My gorgeous friend Laura, whom I mentioned earlier, was getting married to her American fiancé who was a golf pro at that time, and we were travelling over for the wedding. There are so many very funny stories to tell from this trip, Freddie, but I'll give you the edited highlights.

We arrived at the relatively small South Carolina airport at 1 a.m. after a flight from London via Washington, D.C. Being the control freak that I am, I had decided to take charge of booking the condo that we would stay in on Hilton Head Island and the car we would use to get around. I had steeled myself, I was a big girl now, and could manage driving on the right if the car was a good one. We had a discount deal via the BBC so had carefully chosen an SUV Jeep Cherokee – with enough room for us four and our luggage. Feeling pretty tired as we arrived, all of us still just about intact after the scare of a lost passport in Washington (long story!), I got out all my papers from my newly bought and organized travel wallet only to be told by the car-rental check-in clerk that they had run out of SUVs … How can you possibly run out of SUVs? You know how many you have booked in?! So trying to keep my bottom wobbly lip in check, I asked what WAS available … 'A long-wheelbase fifteen-seater van, ma'am' came the super-polite American reply. Well, it seemed we had just two options – to drive the supersize (hey it is America, don't they supersize everything?) vehicle A-Team style – and then some! – or sleep at the airport … and we were four British ladies in desperate need of a snooze. We could pick up the right car from the airport in Hilton Head Island the next day.

Laura had very kindly come out to meet us at the airport to show me how to drive a car with the controls on the steering wheel. Bear in mind she'd only got her own US licence a few weeks before – and I think I'm being fair to say she's never described herself as the best of drivers, – but hey, she was all we had. So I jumped in the driver's side (on the left, Rachael ... remember the left) and Laura showed me the basics of using a stick shift attached to the steering wheel, which felt very odd, while the other girls waited in the car park with our pile of cases. A couple of loops around the top deck of the multi-storey car park and I felt I was ready to nail this. Just one small problem – this van with seats for fifteen people only took two cases. Where is the sense in that? So plenty of room for us to sit, but only a tiny space allocated for luggage. By this point we were losing the will to live, so we rammed our giant 30 kg allowance cases up and over the seats as best we could and we were off to our condo. I did a pretty good job of negotiating our way there safely with much encouragement from the girls. There was just one hairy moment right at the end, where I took a turn into our condo estate and suddenly ended up going the wrong way down the street. There was a lot of shouting from the other girls, but it was about 2 a.m., so we managed to get away with it. The next day I swapped the passenger van for my beloved SUV, never to be bothered by a long wheelbase again!

* * *

We hosted a bachelorette party for Laura just a couple of days later, using foods bought from the delightfully named Piggly Wiggly supermarket. It was not the most refined affair with the conveyor belt of tuna, cheese and egg sandwiches that we had churned out that morning, but it did have slightly melted Jello-O shots brought over by Laura's other bridesmaid that morning, which was my first experience of such a thing. I think the older American ladies that came along were so impressed with the wonderfully English 'Pimms No. 1 Cup' we had brought with us – 'But what is IN it?' 'It's a SECRET, that's the point!' – that we were able to distract them from our slightly shoddy sandwich-making. One thing we did later learn was not to leave out all the leftover buffet overnight with the screendoor open. We woke to a thunderous noise coming from downstairs – Lucy appeared at my door from her neighbouring room, wide-eyed and just repeating the word 'Raccoon?' and we grabbed a broom and cautiously tiptoed into the front lounge to work out where the racket was coming from. It turned out a couple of opportunistic squirrels from the golf course had made their way through the open patio doors and were having a field day at the buffet! We managed to shoo them out, but not before they'd got their grubby little feet over everything and scooted up and down the drapes for good measure. A nice little addition to our clean-up list for that day.

* * *

After eight days of wedding preparations, wedding and wedding tidy-up, us four tired little Welshies were headed for New York, New York! I feel we could have seen it in a better light and that's why I've always wanted to go back in the warm summer months. Unlikely, but I haven't ruled it out yet. As we were only twenty-five and New York hotels are eye-wateringly expensive, we decided to squeeze ourselves into one room with two double beds. If you add in all our winter coats and piles of New York shopping, you can imagine it was quite a feat! Consequently, a few cross words were spoken as we took it in turns in the shower … After nearly two weeks of eating US-sized portions of ribs, fries and burgers, we realized that none of us were as slim as when we'd arrived, so much so we began to get wind burns on our newly acquired muffin tops that were hanging over our jeans in the Big Apple's biting February winds.

Rest assured my Fred, your mummy had many more holidays around the world, exploring new places and collecting memories with lots of friends, Daddy, as well as you! Remember to travel as often as you can, and to always be curious. The world is most definitely your oyster.

Chapter 17

THE BIG C – WHEN CANCER CREPT IN

So, my Freddie, here comes the science bit. The part where I talk about my cancer journey – from being told for the first time what kind of cancer I had, to the different treatments and the surgery. Some moments were really scary and sad, but you know I like to see the funny side where I can, and there are funny bits too – believe it or not!

I hope the amount of science here isn't too much. Cancer is a very complicated disease and, as it turns out, it pays to be fully aware of exactly what it is doing to your body. Each case is individual and in medicine there is no black and white. No one can give you any guarantees. But one thing I know for definite is that I am not a statistic.

Cancer is a big, old, fascinating disease, and some new treatments are cures that are being worked on, so that by the time you're grown up things will be different. Doctors aren't perfect, but they are incredible. They don't stop until they've done everything they can to make you better all round, even if that means you have to wear a freezing cold swimming cap (more on that later) so your hair doesn't fall out or you start to feel like the MRI scanner is your new best friend. The thing is, the cancer I had was a tricky kind, and that's just the luck of the cancer lottery, Fred. You never know what your numbers are going to be. With more research into genetics and cancer, one day doctors will be able to predict your numbers a lot better and more people will make a full recovery more quickly. And that is really good news.

Writing about it in my blog really helped me to accept what was going on and make sense of it all. Knowledge is power. Putting something scary into written words – and talking about it – really does take some of the fear out of it, and not just for the person who's going through it, but also for the people they love and who love them. As terrifying as it is to find out what is going on with your body and that writing it down makes it real, it's much less frightening than keeping it all inside, too scared to admit what is happening to you. The other brilliant thing about talking about something really tough is that you realize you are not alone – I found that out through the blog and the podcast and through all the amazing people I met during my treatment, and let me tell you, that makes a world of difference.

You are so young, and I know you will want your mummy for a long time to come. The thought that you have to grow up without me there to cuddle you when you're sick, after a bad dream or whenever you just want your mummy is too much to bear. It's just not fair. And Freddie, you are so cool and so much fun, I am so annoyed I have to miss out on all the fun times ahead with you! I wanted to include just some of the snippets from my blog, so you can read about Mummy's treatment throughout the different stages, to understand a little bit of what happened and how I was feeling at the time. And remember, it was you and Daddy who kept me strong throughout all of this, and I will be with you always to give you the strength that you need through any tough times.

NOVEMBER 2016

The Beginning

The fortunate thing about a breast cancer diagnosis nowadays is that there is much more awareness of the disease. So women of all ages (and some men, too, as they can also get breast cancer, though much more rarely) are constantly being reminded of the importance of checking their boobs for any unusual signs – such as rashes, changes in size and anomalies on or around the nipples – and of course any lumps that appear, whether in the boobs themselves and also in the armpit area, even if the lump is tiny.

So, I was aware when, one day in the autumn of 2016, I found a lump. Now, most lumps are harmless – they might be cysts or hormonal lumps or sometimes a hair follicle that's got trapped after shaving under the arms – but if you find one, you know you should get it checked out. In my case, I found the lump on a Saturday, saw my GP on the Monday and within three-and-a-half weeks I was diagnosed, biopsied, scanned and sat with my oncologist putting the treatment plan in my diary. She was wonderful and the perfect physician to deal with my overanxiousness and propensity to imagine the worst-case scenario. I instantly trusted her opinions and she met my negative questions with a very jolly dismissiveness.

DECEMBER 2016

The Big C

It's a pretty surreal experience to be told you have cancer. After three hours of tests, the young doctor tasked with delivering the news had her very best 'sorry you have cancer' face on. She kept pausing, waiting for me to cry at opportune moments. I just sat there thinking, 'I wish they'd wrap this up so I can get home, put the baby to bed and watch *I'm a Celebrity*.' I didn't feel I could ask the questions that were burning in my mind, for fear of being thought frivolous. For example, we'd just booked a holiday to Dubai for my birthday in January, and I wondered if we would still be able to go. I did ask the number-one question that was concerning me, though, and I didn't care if it displayed a sense of vanity. Would I lose my hair? Yes, unfortunately was the reply, but it would grow back. That's a difficult thing to digest when you've spent the last few years growing it way past your shoulders. Throughout my adult life I've worn my hair long. I'd always joked that I was a bit like Samson … my strength came from my lion's mane of hair. Well, I was about to find out whether there was any truth in that or if I'd discover that it wasn't the source of my strength …

Triple-Negative

The first biopsy results showed a Grade 3 'triple-negative' tumour, meaning it wasn't a tumour that was receptive to any hormones, and it had also spread to four lymph nodes under my arm. The good news was that a CT scan (a scan of your whole body that shows up cancer where it might be lurking) didn't reveal it to be anywhere else at that moment. It's funny how cancer really lowers your standards of what constitutes good news. After nine days of wondering if I was riddled with the stuff, being told I 'just' had breast cancer felt like a win. Steve and I celebrated with champagne.

Full of post-diagnosis confidence, I decided to consult Dr Google about my type of tumour (I'd previously avoided Googling like the plague, so as not to see anything that would terrify me). Big mistake. The first page I read said that it was more difficult to treat than hormonal-type tumours, more likely to return and had less than five-year survival rate. This sent me into a bit of a tailspin. Steve was away that weekend and my mum was keeping me company. I spent most of the weekend morose and monosyllabic and deep in the depression phase – sorry, Mum! After processing it all with friends and family, I had come to realize that my cancer was just that, mine. My case was not like anyone else's, my outcome would be individual to me. There was no point dwelling on the stats regarding what may come in future.

JANUARY 2017

Chemotherapy

Just like a trip to the dentist, it turns out the anticipation of chemo was worse (for me, anyway) than the reality. After coasting through Christmas, trying to be as normal as possible for all of the family, the dreaded day arrived on 28 December. I kept busy in the morning by going to get my hair cut shorter to be ready for the cold cap (I'll fill you in on the 'horrors of hair' soon), then rushed off to the hospital in time for my appointment. Then we nervously waited … with my imagination going into overdrive about the nightmare to come.

As soon as the familiar face of my lovely chemo nurse appeared, though, I felt okay. We'd met the previous week and she was super upbeat and chipper. She got the whole process started, which began with the cold cap I mentioned earlier. It's basically a hat made up of rubber tubing through which they pump liquid that's been cooled to -5°C. My rough understanding of the science behind it is that the cooling effect prevents the chemo from reaching the hair follicles, which in some cases helps to preserve them and stops the hair from falling out. Getting the cap on proved tricky with Steve nearly (accidentally) punching the lovely chemo nurse in the face in the process. We laughed. It was that kind of delirious laughter you experience while being kept awake all night with a newborn and trying to change a nappy by tag team. Turns out chemo can be funny.

The 'Naughty Drug'

So, head freezing sorted, and after being hooked up to a drip, I was good to go for the chemo drugs, which come in hilariously huge syringes, not unlike something you'd expect to give to a horse. Two that were bright red – 'This is the naughty one, it looks a bit like Tizer,' said my nurse – and then a third which was a different chemo drug that was clear and less scary looking. Then, after a vicious game of Monopoly between Steve and me on the iPad (I won), we were sent on our way with a bag full of drugs and a 'good luck' from the nurses.

By day three, apart from a bit of heartburn and wonky sleep I felt totally normal. So much so that I began to question whether the right drugs had been put in. I did mention it to my nurse – she assured me the drugs would still work. Things got a bit rockier on New Year's Eve and I began to feel a little rougher. My mouth felt pretty weird and my brain felt like a sponge that someone was squeezing the water out of and I was suddenly very, very tired. The kind of tired where you can't even get the muscles in your face to maintain a normal expression. I felt a bit like my face was sagging like the cartoon character Droopy!

But after those two days of grogginess on New Year's Eve and New Year's Day, on 2nd January I woke up feeling pretty normal again and I felt like I'd escaped relatively unscathed so far.

FEBRUARY 2017

Rachael 1 – Chemo 0!

In your face, cancer.

MAY 2017

Lumpectomy

My lumpectomy was scheduled for 19 May, and all went well on the day. I was only in hospital as a day-case, as expected, and the recovery was straightforward. I reacted well to the general anaesthetic as I woke up giddy as a kipper and feeling on top of the world. By the next day, I was in a bit more pain but nothing a few paracetamols couldn't fix. The surgeon told me she'd taken a 'fairly sizeable' area of tissue away but I was in a post 'GA-haze' at the time, so this was quickly forgotten.

Cosmetic Result

As far as the surgery went, it was basically a breast reduction. After one of the male doctors mentioned being 'deformed' afterwards, my hopes for what it would look like were not high! I envisaged being totally lopsided and had looked into padding options. The whole area was very well bandaged, so I couldn't see the results of what was left for a few days. On day five, the surgeon unveiled her work and I was pleasantly surprised with the cosmetic outcome. When I was wearing a bra you really wouldn't notice and that was such a huge psychological boost. I wouldn't normally encourage all and sundry to look at my cleavage, but I was so pleased with the result!

The Recovery

The most painful aspect of the operation was having all the lymph nodes removed from under my arm. It was very sore and afterwards for a while I had to do stretches three times a day to keep the scar tissue flexible. I attracted many a concerned/comedy comment as I leant nonchalantly up against a wall, pulling a pained face while trying to reach my fingertips as high up as possible. For a while I thought my days of throwing a ball for the dog or doing front crawl at the swimming pool were over, but a few weeks on I had almost full movement, though having to carry an enormous bottle around which was attached to a tube that drained excess fluid from under my arm was irritating to say the least. The one evening I knelt on the tubing as I got down on my knees to kiss Freddie goodnight was a particularly low point. I'm afraid his burgeoning vocabulary may have picked up a swear word or two!

Results Day

Then came results day for the post-surgery scan: the moment I'd been dreading. I knew I could still feel a lump there, but I was vainly hoping it was just scar tissue and the tumour was dead inside. The results were delivered by a surgeon I didn't know, as mine was on holiday. They were not what I had hoped. The area of cancer taken out was double the size that had showed up on the scan and one of the margins was 'close'. They look for a minimum of 1mm of cancer-free tissue around the tumour to be happy with the result. While mine was not a positive margin I was told it meant more surgery. I was devastated and had a full-on wailing, teeth-gnashing, fist-clenching breakdown in the car park of the health centre. It felt like after four-and-a-half months of hard work I'd failed the final exam.

Then, just as I picked myself up and came to terms with it, worse news was to come. When I saw my regular surgeon the following week, expecting the new op to be signed off, I was suddenly hit with the news that I would need a mastectomy. I had something called lymphovascular invasion (LVI) around the tumour, which meant the cancer had gone into the lymphatic system of the breast, giving it the ability to spread. I signed the form to have the surgery on the following Friday and left in a daze. I was mentally shattered. It felt like the cracks which cancer had formed in our world were getting bigger and bigger and we'd lost the ability to fix them. One of the worst parts was having to cancel our holiday to Salcombe in Devon (our favourite family spot), which we'd booked at the beginning of the chemo to give ourselves something to look forward to.

But the wonderful thing about the human spirit is that when plunged into the depths of despair, you find your internal warrior takes over and the fighting returns. So, I set about researching all the facts about mastectomy recovery, and through the process of that, a little miracle occurred. After a chat with a surgeon friend of the family – with a view to getting advice on reconstruction options – a question emerged about the kind of cells that were present. From the pathology report it wasn't clear whether they were cancer cells or just the lymphovascular invasion. If it was LVI, that was dealt with by the radiotherapy, NOT by surgery.

A Question

Armed with this information, I went back to my surgeon to ask the difficult question, 'Is this mastectomy needed?' After another chat with the pathologist, it turned out I had a 2mm margin clear of full-blown cancer cells. A much better result, she agreed, and a scenario in which she would never suggest a mastectomy. No further surgery required.

I should add a note here to those of you that I know will be reading this saying, 'If it was me, I'd just want the mastectomy to make sure there was no chance of the cancer coming back'. It's a common misconception that mastectomy eradicates the risk of recurrence. The combination of a lumpectomy and radiotherapy is now accepted as being just effective as a mastectomy. LVI raises the risk of recurrence slightly (by around three per cent over ten years) but very importantly, having a mastectomy does not change this risk. So, in my case it would have been completely unnecessary.

Holiday Time

I was ecstatic. Finally, we had halted the flood of bad news and we left the breast clinic literally kicking our heels and high-fiving each other. The most wonderful part (after not losing a boob) was that our holiday was back on! And another little miracle … our week away coincided with the sun getting his hat on. After the ups and downs of the last few weeks, a week of sunning ourselves on the beautiful beaches around Salcombe was exactly what the doctor ordered.

We returned from holiday refreshed, a bit sunburnt, and ready to face part three. Being signed off for radiotherapy was a lot more of a trial than I thought it would be but, in a weird way, it re-energised me to get through the treatment and out to the other side.

And to add to my celebratory mood, my hair loss hadn't been as bad I was expecting, and it had slowed enough for me to start blow-drying and straightening it again! A trip to the salon for my roots was booked in for a few weeks' time. And the warmer temperatures had encouraged my brows and lashes to grow back with a vengeance. The fog was lifting and I was beginning to feel like my old self again.

JULY 2017

More Bumps in the Road

Just as I was smugly congratulating myself on avoiding a mastectomy and admiring my new radiotherapy tattoos, a call one evening from my breast-care nurse threw everything into uncertainty again. My latest CT scan, while clear everywhere else, had shown up some 'areas of concern' in the same breast we thought we'd just rid of cancer.

My breast-care nurse hugged me on the way in and the surgeon had on her 'bad-news head-tilt', so I prepared myself for bad news. Good news: one of the biopsies had just showed inflammation. Bad news: the other showed more cancer, in a new area of the breast. That mastectomy I thought I'd so cleverly avoided was actually needed. If it's got to go, it's got to go, I thought. If that was what it took for me to be able to stick around and see my Fred go off to university one day, then I was gladly going to give it up to the cause.

Muddy Waters

Exactly what had been going on in my body was unclear. Had this new cancer sprung up during and post chemotherapy? Or was it always there and just missed because I didn't have the right scans? The tumour never even showed up on a mammogram in the beginning despite being obvious on an ultrasound scan. I choose to believe that it was just hidden on the scan, which would also explain why the area of cancer that was taken out in my lumpectomy was twice the size to what had showed up on the ultrasound. It feels more comforting to think it was always just hiding out there, rather than a crazily aggressive cancer that was growing quickly. We'll never know for sure, as I was never given an MRI scan at the start to properly image what was going on. The waters had become so muddied I rather lost faith in the process, so went for a second opinion. I decided to switch doctors and hospitals as the doctor/patient relationship couldn't really function without full trust. All this has led us to the door of a mastectomy which happened in late July.

AUGUST 2017

Groundhog Day

The pathology results from the mastectomy surgery knocked me for six again, as it turned out that another, bigger and badder tumour had been lurking in the breast that was removed. My scar had literally just healed from the mastectomy – already my second operation – so to be told it was back to the operating table for the third time was frustrating to say the least. I so thought that the chemo had done its job and we were cruising to the finish line, only for me to veer off course and get lost somewhere along the way (I've always had a TERRIBLE sense of direction). But was just going to have to reset the sat-nav and get us to our destination via a diversionary route.

So, more chemo. My oncologist called to tell me this while I was sat in the hairdresser's chair with a head full of foils getting the highlights and blow dry I'd been waiting eight months for. The irony was almost worthy of an Alanis Morissette lyric! Another eighteen weeks of an all-out ban on germs and hair straighteners. I was told the two new drugs I'd be given wouldn't cause too much hair loss, possibly just a bit of thinning. I hoped to 'cold cap' again, even if it meant avoiding just a five per cent loss. I wasn't prepared to give up another hair on my head to this disease. HOWEVER, THE THREAT OF MORE CHEMO COULDN'T TAKE AWAY THE JOY OF MY FIRST COLOUR AND BLOW DRY IN EIGHT MONTHS!

The New Plan

After the chemo, I was fast-tracked onto my radiotherapy. During the treatment I entertained myself, while trying to lay as still as possible, by imagining Dr Evil's voice asking the radiographers to 'Set the frickin' lasers'. It was all fun.

Then I got a three-week break before another eighteen weeks of chemo. After some 'initial resistance' (i.e. wailing and crying and shouting 'Why me?!?!'), I steeled myself for it. It meant my fortieth birthday in January would be spent in the chemo suite rather than on the slopes of the Alps as I'd planned! The finish line may have moved, but our resolve to reach it had not …

OCTOBER 2017

Expect the Unexpected

From the moment I was diagnosed with breast cancer, the fear of recurrence was something that occupied a lot more of my headspace than it should have. But I hadn't thought for a moment that we wouldn't be able to get rid of it the first time. Yet ten months into treatment, here I was about to embark on a second lot of chemo in the space of a year – I'd drawn the short straw and got the cancer equivalent of being seated next to the dull bloke at dinner. It's tedious, boring, goes on *waaaay* too long and takes you away from all the fun stuff you could be doing instead.

I developed an excellent ability to pretend this wasn't happening for much of the time. But all too often, usually when my mind was not well occupied enough, in came … THE FEAR. It wasn't always a source of misery. Sometimes it raised a laugh, like the time I asked Steve if he thought I'd be worthy of an 'all BBC Staff email' if I died. I really was only half joking … But even when we're laughing together and having fun, THE FEAR can strike, like when I suddenly think how awful it would be for Steve to be left without anyone to chuckle over in-jokes with. He doesn't deserve that.

CT Scan

Then, the day after starting the second round of chemo, I chased up the results of the scan I'd had a few weeks before, thinking blithely that all would be fine as they'd call if something showed up, right? Wrong. I was told to come in that day to speak to the oncologist. All I could think after coming off the phone was, 'I don't want to go, I don't want to go'.

The scan had showed an enlargement of the lymph nodes under the arm on the OPPOSITE side to my original cancer. This was a very unusual place for it to go to (more common is the brain, liver, lungs or bones) but hey, why change the habit of a lifetime? My cancer only does weird and unusual. Technically, this meant the cancer had metastasized – travelled away from its primary site – and that made me stage 4. Which was bad.

NOVEMBER 2017

Coping With It

When people asked how I coped with it all, I told them it could never be as bad as getting my first set of pathology results six months prior. I was inconsolable after having all my hopes of chemo doing a good job dashed with the news that the cancer they'd taken out was bigger that what they'd thought was there in the first place. That's not to say I'd lost hope. I just kept it a little better protected from blows being rained down from this prize fighter of a cancer.

Living in Hope

Please don't think I stopped fighting. I'd worked every bit as hard as those whose cancer has been treated successfully. I'd just been unfortunate to pick the big scoring card in the Top Trumps of cancer. It felt like I'd been thrown back down to the bottom of the mountain of treatment again. But my only option was to keep climbing, as I knew how beautiful the view was from the top.

A Plan

Things were looking a bit more positive since my last post and there was now a plan in place. As ever there was a bit of disagreement, it wouldn't feel right if *everything* was nailed down! The mid-chemo CT scan showed the nodes under my arm to be stable, with one possibly a little smaller. The chemo *was* working, in that they weren't growing, but it wasn't smashing them, so we decided to finish at four rounds and go to surgery. Annoyingly though, they discounted the first round I had with the different drug combination (one that tried to give me a heart attack – I know, seriously!) so it meant there was still another round to go. Just in time for my fortieth …

I kind of wanted to rush through Christmas and get into January because after a little more chemo, I could be having my surgery by the start of February and finally felt like I was ridding myself of the last cells of this crappy cancer. The sooner the surgery was done, the sooner I could get on with my plans for the new year of getting back on the ski slopes (I'd even got a fancy new ski jacket from Steve for Christmas as a placeholder) and running (mostly walking!) the London Marathon for Macmillan in April.

DECEMBER 2017

Merry Chemo Christmas!

I started my chemo on 28 December last year and guess where I'd be exactly one year on? Yep, on the chemo ward. It had been a pretty horrendous year, but by no means all bad. I'd made some brilliant new friends, and had also started and grown my blog, 'Big C. Little Me'.

We'd agreed a new plan for my treatment, and when it was put in place I had a new sense of purpose to get through the next few months. So, I wished very much for a Merry Christmas for all of us and a brighter and less cancery new year!

MARCH 2018

Bad News

I'm sorry I didn't write for a while, but we had a difficult few months. I so hoped that things could have been more positive, but unfortunately the bad news kept on racking up. My lymph node surgery in February went to plan, but the results as ever weren't good. Seven out of nineteen nodes removed were positive for cancer – a sign the previous four months of chemo hadn't really cut the mustard. Still, my surgeon was happy he'd done as much as he could, and a subsequent scan a couple of weeks later showed no new nasty surprises. Though troublingly, a spot on my hip that they'd been monitoring had grown slightly. Still, no reason to be reaching for the lifeboats just yet.

APRIL 2018

You, Me and the Big C Podcast

I was back at work five days a week and having so much fun doing our new *You, Me and the Big C* podcast, with my beautiful and fabulous new friends, Deborah James and Lauren Mahon. I was making sure I did all my post-surgery stretches, but after a few weeks I became aware that my breast on the latest surgery side was a little swollen. Still no bells started to ring. Then it started to go red. I presumed lymphoedema had set in – a very annoying but not dangerous condition where lymph fluid collects after nodes have been removed. But it obviously looked a bit odd as the lymphoedema team sent me back to the surgeon. Then the sirens started to wail. Biopsies were taken. The surgeon's demeanour was serious. Fingers were crossed.

APRIL 2018

The Call

I got the call when I was out at the ice-cream farm with Freddie and some of his little pals. My heart raced as I answered it, knowing a phone call did not bode well. Then came the words 'I am so sorry, it's bad news. The biopsies have come back showing the same cancer is back and is in the skin.' I watched my little Freddie innocently playing away in a tyre in the barn and my heart broke for him. I scooped him up and dashed home and then had to break Steve's heart with the news that my cancer was now metastatic and therefore incurable.

Waiting

There was a lot of waiting. First for a grim-faced meeting with the oncologist. I turned up a little hopeful, thinking that at least by the time we left we'd have a plan, even if that was just to extend things for a while. Action always feels good. But he explained – as if I didn't know it all too well already – that my cancer hadn't responded well to chemo thus far. And with chemo there's usually no magic button;

we wouldn't suddenly find one that smashed it. So, I was told my best chance for extra time was with treatment with a 'novel agent'. I had to ask what that was, as images of James Bond flashed through my head. It basically meant a brand-new drug, something fresh and innovative that was in the early stages of trial and development. I was referred to the Clinical Trials Unit in Manchester. There was more waiting, all the while watching and feeling the cancer spread.

JUNE 2018

Frontier of Science

So, this was where we were: I had extensive skin metastases in my left breast and chest, mets to the nodes above the collarbone on the left side, a tumour in my liver and a couple of suspicious spots on my spine. I also had a small collection of fluid on the outside of my right lung called a pleural effusion, which was indicative of some cancer starting to lurk there. So that was skin, nodes, liver, bones, lung. I think even the unscientific among you could do the math on that one.

I started on the first clinical trial they had in store for me. It worked by getting your own immune system to start attacking the cancer. It performed well in some types of cancer, but not in breast cancer. If it didn't help me, then I hoped the data I provided would at some point in the future help others in the same position.

JULY 2018

More Bad Results

I headed into the Christie Hospital in Manchester for my scan results full of trepidation. On clinical trials you generally live or die (excuse the pun) by how the results inform the doctors. I asked if I was having an electrocardiogram (ECG) and the nurse told me that no, it wasn't written on her sheet. But I knew from the trial schedule that if things were on track, then I should have been taken for an ECG. Red flag.

Every time I was there and having my observations done, I'd have to take a little walk around the corridors to see if my oxygen sats went up after a little exercise. As I passed the waiting room and saw Steve down the corridor, I shook my head at him. He could see from my expression that things were not going to go well.

The Green Mile

Then I got put in the consulting room to wait for my doctor, by now feeling like I was walking the medical equivalent of the Green Mile. My doctor arrived … with the trial nurse in tow. Another bad sign, as normally it's just the doc. First the one bit of good news: it was the first time I'd had my head scanned and nothing was showing in the brain.

But it was all downhill from there. The main killer headline was my liver lesion, which had grown by more than the twenty per cent allowed. Quite significantly more, in fact, and that meant I was not allowed to continue on the trial as it could cause liver failure.

The most problematic areas at that time were my lungs, which were quite frankly a bit of a mess. I hadn't been able to breathe well under any exertion for weeks by that point. My poor little lungs were basically crumpled up like a ball of paper at the top of my chest. I was still doing a bit of work and podcasting, though, and going to all the amazing events my fairy-godmother friends had got me tickets for.

A scan showed that my lungs were gradually sucking up fluid like sponges and severely hampering my ability to breathe. They put me on some steroids to try and calm the situation. My reaction – 'I don't want to be fat and have a moon-face'! Then overnight things deteriorated somewhat, as I woke up every hour totally out of breath and just knowing that I needed oxygen. Add to that chills and a high temperature, and I was snatching the steroids out of their hands.

Going Backwards

After another two nights in Hotel Christie, I was sent home in an ambulance on oxygen and was given steroids by the bucket-load, swallowing them along with my vain worries about dying fat! An oxygen machine was installed at home. I hated it. It was noisy and a sign of the creeping medicalization of our home that I had watched happen when my dad died. It had an incredibly long plastic tube attached to it, so I could move around the house and garden. Anytime a toddler, dog or family member trod on it my head would whip back like Beyoncé in full swing.

So, the lowdown was that they had one more trial left for me at the Christie. I had already pre-screened and had the necessary mutation required to take part. But any respiratory issues had to be stable. That meant not being on oxygen and not having my lungs fill up with fluid again. I managed a full day without extra oxygen the day before, so now I just needed my lungs to stay fluid free over the next week. The doctors said we just 'need a few days of stability' for me to be able to sign up. I was due to see them tomorrow, for which I'd have my best game face on. I thought, 'Let's do this'.

Reflecting on Friendship

This brings me to – without doubt – the positive part of having cancer: the joy, gratitude and strength you feel from the support of those around you, like the old friends I'd lost touch with, who sent me some beautiful and inspiring messages. To feel so many people pulling for you is good. You need that when facing tough times coming up. As a people pleaser, I didn't want to let them down. I knew I had to do this and get out the other side.

I received flowers and gifts, and each one with its accompanying message made me cry. I was just floored by the kindness and generosity of people. I'm so used to giving myself a hard time, I hadn't stopped to think that the rest of the world wasn't always doing the same. One fabulous friend sent me a gorgeous cashmere robe … and the note with it read 'When the going gets tough … the tough get cashmere'. It's a mantra I now plan to live my life by. One that Steve quickly started rueing.

Then there are the complete strangers, the cancer survivors I was put in touch with, who'd taken the time to talk me through their experiences and give me advice on everything they'd learnt. They saved me a lot of Googling by sending me tips, lists and forums on how to survive the chemo, the surgery, the recovery, the guilt and the fear. They were there when the road got rocky and they knew that sometimes you don't want to be positive and you just need a good cry. To see so many people are still smiling is such a wonderful source of hope.

My oldest friends were amazing. They immediately set up a fundraising page to get money together for a wig. I was never going to be rocking an NHS synthetic number. It had to be real human hair all the way for me and looking as close to my natural style as possible. Vain? Possibly. But as I read on one cancer website ... vanity is sanity! It was such a wonderful gesture – trying to look vaguely normal with cancer is an expensive business! I was blown away by the generosity of people, from old schoolfriends I'd not seen in years to complete strangers I'd never met. All of these wonderful people helped to make me that little bit stronger, ready for the fight ahead.

Family Support

Along with my fabulous friends, I'm very lucky to have a wonderful family support network around me. I know if someone has to go through this, then I'm as good a person as any, as I have such a great team. Steve is of course the Captain. One of our friends, on hearing the news, sent a message saying that if you ever had to go through cancer, then Steve would be the man you'd want alongside you. It had been only a few years since our beautiful wedding, when we were so full of hope for what our future together would hold. We stood at the front of that church and promised to love each other in sickness and in health. Neither of us could have imagined the sickness part would come so soon. I felt terribly guilty that he was having to go through this because of me. That's apparently quite common among women with cancer.

But he told me so many times that he'd rather go through cancer with me than have an easy time with anyone else. So, he's been there for every appointment, holding my hand and picking me up when

I've been down. I still feel bad that has picked up a lot of slack on the days I'm feeling rough, when I can't be able to pull my weight with the childcare and household chores. It now seems fortuitous that I've always been a really dreadful housewife – because me being out of action isn't be such a wrench to him! I don't cook and I only clean sporadically. I told him I'd actually just had him in training through our marriage so far, ready for this moment when he'd need to fully grab the reins of domestic drudgery. Well, young Jedi, your time has come. Let's hope I don't get too out of practice that I never pick up a duster again! I was incredibly lucky with the support of Steve, the whole family and my brilliant friends, they made the whole process as simple as it could be.

* * *

SEPTEMBER 2018

Freddie, your daddy and I said we would leave no stone unturned in the search to fix this cancer and we did our best. We kept up with all of what was going on in my treatment – I was very much my own patient advocate as I think it's important to at least understand your medical position on a basic level in order to make decisions regarding your treatment plan. As per usual I went one step beyond and researched a bit more than most, but my situation was a complex one. Many friends said I could be an oncologist with all the cancer information I'd learnt – I was only joking when I said there wasn't much more to know!

From the very start of my cancer journey, this was no fair fight. It was grade 3 – the highest in terms of cells growing and dividing. It started as stage 3 – as high as it can get without technically becoming metastatic. I had triple-negative breast cancer – so there were no conventional post-treatment drugs like your hormonally driven Herceptin and

Tamoxifen. When my treatment 'finished', I never got months of time off thinking I was in remission. I knew there were always some nasty little cells lurking about in there waiting to catch me out again. But I thought I was ready to catch them out.

But the last moment came when the grim-faced oncologist delivered the very grimmest of news this week, a job I did not envy him one bit. Dr Sacha Howell had a long history at the Christie in Manchester – his father before him had worked in the research department – and you know if this man is telling you that there's nothing more they can do, then he isn't joking. But the real blow came when I asked, 'How long?' – something I'd been reluctant to put a number on before – and the answer came back 'Days … possibly weeks'. That was such a shock – one that, as I write this, we've not quite dealt with yet. Daddy says that's all he keeps hearing going around in his head. We thought we were quite up on our 'death admin' but suddenly pensions needed forms, 'i's needed dotting and 't's crossing, and most of all I wanted to finish this book for you, my darling. That's the most important part. Freddie, I so hope you can pick up on all the advice that I've dropped throughout this book.

Chapter 18

A MOTHER'S LOVE

My beautiful son. I so wish that I didn't have to leave you now. But believe me I tried EVERYTHING I could to stay around for you for every moment I could eke out of this life. I'm sure some of the press and media will say I 'lost my battle with cancer'. I didn't, that's just lazy journalism – I didn't lose anything. From the outset it was not a fair fight with this cancer. My cancer was too big and too aggressive and we didn't begin on a level playing field. You were fourteen months old and at the very start I was so full of fierce intention that we could get past this. I would lay you in your cot each night and communicate from my mind to yours, 'I will do this, Freddie. I will take whatever they have to throw at me and I will take it gladly if it means we can still stay together.' Then as you grew and began to talk and interact more, that unspoken mantra became a more vocal one and I would hug you and squeeze you every night, promising you out loud for the universe to hear that I would do this for us. And I NEVER stopped trying, not for a moment.

Over the last few years a real vapid culture of superficiality has arisen, particularly aimed at young people. I'm talking the Kar-trashian gang and their followers. Or their Towie equivalents in the UK – they make huge amounts of money from doing very little but peddling their merchandise. Look around you for the true beauty in the natural world. I've already told you about checking up to the stars which Mummy loves and looking for Mummy there.

Give back to the people who give to you, look for those who may need your help – give without expecting anything back. Life can be short or long – every second is precious so make it count.

Freddie, part of the reason for writing this book was that so you could know me almost as well as if I was still there with you. I hope you don't mind me sharing all of this – it was done with every good intention. I also hope Daddy has filled you in on plenty more stories from our wonderful time together. It might have been short but I promise you, my darling boy, that it was filled with fun and adventure. Just as with the cancer treatment, we left no stone unturned. We loved, we laughed, we cried, and we did it all together. As a family.

And I also trust that Daddy has passed on to you some of my most treasured possessions, like my beautiful engagement ring, which brought me so much joy, and my wedding ring, placed on my finger by Daddy on the most special of days. Hopefully I have left enough behind for you to feel me with you everywhere you go.

Be kind. Be good. Be strong. Be true, my Freddie. I know you have the most wonderful life ahead of you. And know through it all that your mummy loves you with every last tiny piece of her heart. You're not even three yet but people say you are the spitting image of me and I know that will always give Daddy comfort. I so desperately wanted to see you grow up – as I've already said, I get terrible FOMO, and as I write this, that is perhaps the most painful thing because I know we would have had such fun together.

You will always be the most special of boys – we remain the Three Best Friends wherever I am in the ether. All my love to you always.

Mummy x

Rachael Bland

B. 21 January 1978 – D. 5 September 2018

Chapter 19

MEMORIES OF MUMMY

Tony Livesey

As I write this I'm sitting next to Rachael's desk at BBC Radio 5 Live. Before our *Drive* show together we'd often put the world to rights from this position, and when she was diagnosed with cancer we often discussed how medical science might put her right too. It wasn't to be.

As time passed and Rachael began to come to terms with her diagnosis, she asked me one day what I thought of the idea that she might write a book for her son, Freddie; it was to be full of her memories, her dreams, her likes and dislikes. Essentially, it was to be full of Rachael. You now hold it in your hands.

I've been asked to write a few words for it. I originally said those words, proudly and emotionally, in the eulogy I gave at Rachael's funeral. After the service her mum told me that Rachael called me her 'radio husband'. So … for my radio wife, here's what I felt at the time and feel even more strongly as the days go by.

The Eulogy

I can't remember exactly what night it happened as Rachael and I presented the late show on 5 Live together, nine years or so ago. Perhaps it was the night I was asking listeners what was the last thing that fell on their head? Maybe it was the time I was asking people how far they'd travelled in their slippers? Or was it the show when I was asking for stories about encounters with wildlife and a listener rang in to say he'd woken up that morning and found a slug on his wife's bottom? Anyway, it was during one of those award-winning moments that Rachael invented her catchphrase: 'Shall we move on?'

I can't tell you how many times, using that very line, that she probably saved my career. Actually, she loved playing the faux schoolmistress, an upstairs to my downstairs, the voice of sanity who secretly loved to lose it.

I paid her back in style. She was allowed to turn on the first official 5 Live foghorn at South Shields – with a plummy 'Switch orn the foghorn!' And when we recreated the *Coronation Street* tram crash – with the actual driver – she was given a speaking role on the tram. If I remember correctly, her line was 'Aaaaaagh!' Whatever we threw at Rachael, as you would imagine, she more than coped.

Above everything, she was a supreme professional. It was only after her death that I learnt in an on-air interview with the station boss that Rachael – in the nicest possible way – actually wanted to stay with Richard Bacon on his new show rather than team up with me. I've tweeted recently about how she metaphorically held my hand as I made my radio debut. It's testament to Rachael's professionalism that she didn't let it show for a minute that, rather than holding my hand, she'd actually been cuffed to it!

Notwithstanding how we became co-presenters, we quickly became friends; and so, like all of you, I got to know a remarkable woman. That smile. That openness. That warmth. That pragmatism. That cheeriness. That determination. And once you knew her, that vulnerability which was lightly worn. That tolerance, too.

On the occasions when I was mid-flight of fancy or teasing her or being profoundly ridiculous, the listeners used to text to say they could hear Rachael rolling her eyes in exasperation. She got her revenge in style. On the night that 5 Live officially moved to Salford, I was chosen to be the first voice on air. It was a prestigious moment. They printed posters. The bigwigs were up from London and staring at me through the glass. I'd crafted my first words – Churchillian, they were. Just as I drew breath, Rachael waltzed into the studio, sat down and read the news. Hers was the first voice. I, naturally, was absolutely seething. We laughed afterwards and I'm so glad now that Rachael has her place in 5 Live history.

Conversely, she fluffed her own official big moment. She was due to announce the winner of the 2010 Mercury Prize in a piece of breaking news, but was bamboozled by a reference to 'The xx' in the script. She thought the producer had put in the random letters 'xx' as a placeholder until the winner was known, but 'The xx' was actually the name of the award-winning band. 'I can't bring you that news about who won the Mercury Prize,' Rachael informed her listeners, 'but I will hopefully before the end of this bulletin …' She powered through as she always did.

She went on to present *Up All Night* among other shows, before we were reunited to present *Drive* every Friday. And boy, did she shine. She was witty when required – I already knew she could be that – but when news was breaking, chaos was ensuing and serious issues had to be dealt with quickly, incisively and accurately, she was effortless in that professionalism I've already described.

She was that one thing we all strive to be when the news is tough, hard to listen to but necessary to deliver – 100 per cent reliable.

And that was the approach she brought to coping with cancer. Rachael was determined to be a rock for Freddie and Steve. For months before each Friday show we'd chat about her illness, her progress, her fears and, yes, her desperation as the treatments became trials and hope began to fade.

The only time she ever privately expressed any concern to me was about how they'd cope without her. I was determined to encourage her to write her book for Freddie. Rachael knew my circumstances – my mum died from cancer when I was thirteen – so asked how I thought Freddie would feel to read about her in a book available to all. I said put down every word, every thought, every like, every dislike, every single thing you've felt and done. He'll be grateful for every word and proud that other people can share.

When Rachael died I wrote that the closer she came to death, her determination to stick two fingers up to this bloody disease became gloriously disproportionate to the state of her health. She defied a conventional death and it turns out she took the whole country along for the ride.

An illustration of that is the fact that a very good friend of mine has just finished her chemo and radiotherapy to treat breast cancer, and throughout all of this she and Rachael swapped emails. But that's not all. My friend texted me last night to say a friend of hers is sadly in the final stages of cancer. Let's call him John. John's family sent a message out to all his friends and part of it said this …: 'I urge you to go to the podcast *You, Me and the Big C* and download the episode "About Death". It is beautiful and comforting. I played it to John and the girls and they have found it of great comfort. John would like you to know he has come to terms with things and is not afraid to die and hopes this is of comfort to you all.' Rachael, Deborah, Lauren – job done, I reckon.

Rachael has left some legacy. As I said on the day she died, in her selfless determination that others should benefit from her crappy predicament, she broke taboos, raised spirits, laughed in the face of cancer and gave us a right rollocking if we didn't laugh with her.

So, on that basis, and in conclusion, I'd like to introduce you to the third person in our relationship. It's not Steve, not Freddie, not even Richard Bacon. It's a certain Randy Bumgardener. We were being daft again on lates, asking 'Who on earth would want to be called Randy?' As ever, listeners joined in and mentioned US politician Randy Bumgardener. It was Rachael's job to announce this – and around 200,000 people have listened to what happened subsequently just over the past few days. When you hear this clip, Rachael can't help herself near the start and either tells me or herself off, I'm not sure which, when she says between her infectious giggles, 'Sorry, I'm so childish!'

But it's the laugh I want to hear again. The laugh I'll never forget. The laugh before cancer. The laugh which is beautifully natural before she was put through hell.

We won't remember the cold cap, the dreadful diagnosis, the fear, the tears, the black cloud that tried to blight her life. Instead, you can find the clip online via this web link: www.bbc.co.uk/programmes/p06kg2nm/. Enjoy one minute and thirty-five seconds of pure Rachael. That laugh, though!

Richard Bacon

There are many reasons why Rachael was so special. Not least because, in the teeth of her terminal diagnosis, she produced the greatest work of her life: the podcast, *You, Me and the Big C*, and the book you are holding in your hands right now.

I worked with Rachael quite a lot. Chiefly on the late-night show on BBC Radio 5 Live. We began each evening at 10 p.m., a very nice time to be on the radio, and ended at 1 a.m., a not very nice time to be on the radio. So we invented an ironically named club, the 'Special Half Hour', to lazily fill up the last bit of the show when we'd usually get bored. It was made up mainly of the 'William Tell Overture', unexplained appearances from Quentin Willson and Rachael reading out emails from listeners claiming that this club was the most important thing that had ever happened to them.

Out of this silliness stood Rachael. She had this ability to effortlessly switch from earnest news to nonsense. From information to complete irreverence. Just weeks in, a dedicated, obsessive 'Rachael Bland Fan Club' sprang up with thousands of subscribers. Such was the impact she had had on their lives that eight years after the show had ended and thus the club had folded, some of its former members came to pay their respects at her funeral. The qualities we saw during those late nights, Rachael would go on to refine and use with pioneering brilliance in her final months.

To quote her husband Steve, 'When her body was at its weakest, her voice was at its strongest'. And so she produced the famous podcast and this book, *For Freddie*. Both are frank and witty, sometimes shocking, always breezy. Surprising, original and joyful. The Rachael you will read in these pages, the Rachael on air, the Rachael in the podcast and Rachael in real life are all *exactly* the same. Which is another way of saying she was truly natural.

Her death brutally reminded me of things that, of course, I already knew. Cancer is cruel and unjust and in its closing stages, quick. The end made me see things I wish I'd seen before. We underestimated her. We only noticed just how talented she was as the clock was running down. But still, she proved her point.

Rachael said of Freddie, 'It feels like he's at an age where he might not even have any memories of me … so I'm writing down my whole life in a book for him and I just hope through his life he will come back to that book … and feel like he knows the kind of person his mother was.' A lovely idea, of course, and he *will* see that in this book.

He will also grow up and listen to the podcasts and read the tributes and he will know not just that his mum was courageous, funny, authoritative, clever and a great laugh, but that she was loved by all of us who knew her, and by many thousands of people who never even met her. You will have noticed in the earlier pages of the book that, despite being ill during the writing process, she comes across as natural and as vibrant and as full of life as ever. Just as she was in the years before the Big C got anywhere near her. And that is how I will remember her. She was brilliant.

Jonathan Wall

I was Rachael's boss for five years, and she was a dear colleague of mine for sixteen years. She was funny, charming and very bright.

In her twenties she was already one of the country's finest newsreaders. Not long after, she became an essential part of 5 Live's late-night radio – first with Richard Bacon and then with Tony Livesey.

Her presenting developed further – and emboldened by both marriage and motherhood she clicked into another gear, demonstrating a blend of warmth and authority behind the microphone. And all of that is before we even talk about the podcast. In her own right she had already become a great broadcaster, and then sometimes projects and opportunities come along that turn those great people into heroic people.

When she first approached me with the idea of the podcast I knew it was something she was capable of pulling off. I had real concerns, though, knowing that some of the scan results hadn't been going to plan. Would this be something too challenging emotionally to pull off if she grew poorly quite quickly? I underestimated her incredible courage and determination to help others. She created the finest work of her life in the final year of her life. Her real legacy is, of course, the beautiful Freddie and the way she has enhanced the lives of all of those who knew her.

The podcast, though, is a wonderful professional legacy and we at 5 Live are determined to see *You, Me and the Big C* grow from strength to strength.

Emma Barnett

What I liked immediately about Rachael was her honesty and bluntness. If I'm honest myself, I was quite intimidated by her during our first meeting, as she sat down, cool as a cucumber, to read the news on my new BBC Radio 5 Live programme. I thought I had somehow offended her. It turned out she had recently discovered that she had cancer and was finishing up one of her initial rounds of treatment.

I soon became an avid reader of her erudite blog and in our snatched moments – between the mic light flashing red – appreciated the no-nonsense way she updated me on her progress and hopes. These dispatches were delivered swiftly, without self-indulgence and while she disinfected all of the equipment she needed in our studio. Every. Single. Bulletin. She took it all in her stride.

I was honoured when she chose to talk to me on air about her cancer journey and the toll her treatment was taking. Our listeners loved Rach – they really did – as evidenced by the texts, calls and tweets that avalanched in after each time she shared the latest part of her experience.

When we posed for a photo after one of our interviews, she styled it in the short time we had between links. I was to stand on her right, as she knew her better side and wanted it captured accordingly. I laughed and uncharacteristically did as I was told. And that was Rach – charming, straightforward and with a keen grasp of what needed to be done.

I miss her voice, warmth and our banter – alongside our millions of listeners.

Rachel Burden

Rachael and I worked together for many years and in many ways our paths intertwined. She was the brilliant, elegant journalist sitting alongside me in the studio; she was a woman establishing a strong and articulate voice in what was still sometimes a very male world; she was a young mother battling sleep deprivation yet still word-perfect (unlike me) on the radio; she was a fellow girl about town in Knutsford where we both lived, clinking glasses and spending joyful times with her friends.

Losing Rachael deeply affected us all. She was so healthy, beautiful and strong – we are now all so aware of the fragility of life. She loved her boy with absolute ferocity and we all now cling on a little longer to our own babies. In the darkest of days, she shone so brightly and squeezed every last bit of goodness out of the life she had left – may we all live a little better because of her. Through her podcast she pushed radio boundaries and gave enormous comfort to others, and we are all now a little braver about talking about cancer and dying.

I'm so glad Freddie will know Rachael a little better through this book. She was a wonderful woman but most of all a wonderful mother, Freddie, and she'll never be forgotten.

Mark Pougatch

Whenever Rachael came into the studio to read the news – amid a normal, faintly hectic 5 Live sports programme – she always brought with her total professionalism, calmness and authority, but just as importantly a sense of humour and a twinkle in her eye such that you could throw anything at her, in any subject, and she'd respond in an entertaining way.

But for all that gravitas as a newsreader, she will rightly always be remembered for opening up the nation's conversation about cancer and terminal illness. What she, Deborah and Lauren have done is quite remarkable. They have challenged us to talk about cancer in a matter-of-fact manner and not hide behind opaque language.

I went to the first talk that Deborah and Lauren did after Rachael's death. It was striking how many people there – of both sexes and a range of ages – were cancer sufferers who were so open in talking about their illness and their fears. It was both a sad and yet uplifting evening. Bless you, Rachael.

Greg Wise

I never met Rachael in person, but I shared an incredibly powerful time with her only weeks before she died – she in a radio studio in Salford, and me, alongside Deborah and Lauren in London, recording for their *You, Me and the Big C* podcast.

We had an extraordinary conversation – open and searingly honest. Rach was able to assume her role in the vanguard, as the pioneer – trailblazing this subject that usually makes people mute, with an honesty and compassion. She was bearing witness. Always with a spark of humour to soften the blow – 'I'm your "It could be worse" person. I like to provide a service.' But, also acutely aware that often others cannot take her japing – 'My death jokes are bombing at the moment.'

Oddly, we feel that we need to protect those we love from our death – and not talking about it is a loving gesture. But it is actually, I think, cruel. Talking about death is an act of love. And in the time I spent talking with Rachael, I witnessed a profound love – not just for Steve and Freddie, not just for Deborah and Lauren, but for everybody. She was, after all, a broadcaster – wanting to get to the essence of a story, and to try and translate that to her listeners. This is what she did at this most painful, and possibly most personal, of times. Using what she was discovering to help others who maybe aren't as brave as she was, to be able to bring this subject out into the sunlight – to cleanse, to detoxify death. She was able to create, in that radio studio, an almost spiritual space – a confessional. She said, 'It's not the dying process that gives me any fear – it's the leaving people behind.'

At the end of the podcast, Rach talks about a book she wants to write for her son, Freddie. Having now achieved that goal, she has ensured that Freddie will be able to learn what a brave, honest, human and funny person his mum was – able to stand squarely in the face of her own death and give testament as her final act of love.

Shelagh Fogarty

I'm on a train from London to Liverpool to see my mum. I do it most weekends these days because I love her to bits, she is easy to spend time with and she needs me and my siblings a bit more now she is what the Irish call 'a great age'. I love that expression because it feels celebratory, grand and full of respect.

When Rachael died, Mum and I discussed how very sad it is that a young mother won't get to experience all the aspects of her child's life from that moment on and he won't have her either. Bette Davis wasn't wrong when she said, 'Growing old is not for cissies', though she might easily have added, 'but I'll take it over dying young'.

Rachael has died too young. Plain and simple. It does not seem fair or right, but there it is. Steve and Freddie have to live in that world now, and as much as I'm writing this for Rachael I'm doing it for them really, and especially Freddie, to help him when he is older to rebuild, inadequately of course, what he has lost.

So, Freddie, in lots of ways your mummy was like mine. Gentle, ladylike, concerned her hair looked right and utterly devoted to her beautiful child. In the first picture of you that she sent me you were about three months old. In it, you're nestled in her legs and she is taking the photo as you look up to her. It struck me then and it does now that it's an image of pure mother love captured for ever in your huge smile as you gaze back at her. I doubt she was ever happier, and I doubt you were ever safer or more loved than in that moment. You still had plenty more such moments to come until the clouds gathered, but they can never be lost, Fred. She is in every cell of your body and every fibre of your heart, so see! You do still have her.

Not a great age, but a great, great mother who has left you everything you need.

Deborah James

Rachael was one of my best friends. She taught me how to die and, by doing so, taught me how to live. I couldn't be prouder to have been a part, albeit a short part, of her life. In 2016, just before Christmas, both of us were trying to make sense of the hands we had been dealt. The words 'You have cancer' had come crashing into our lives and everything stopped. I was a thirty-five-year-old deputy head teacher with stage 4 bowel cancer. She was a marathon-running broadcaster with breast cancer.

We met through blogging – we wanted to share our stories not only to help us to process the situation, but also to let others know that they were not alone. We bonded over a gritty determination to do something productive. Our motto was 'Get busy living in the hope dying will wait'. And, for me, Rachael became the person I could turn to in the middle of the night and ask: 'Are you scared too?'

When she was diagnosed in 2016, Rachael was in her prime. Jonathan Wall, controller of Radio 5 Live, described her as one of the best presenters under forty at the BBC. Her career ranged from news to drivetime to breakfast shows. When her life was turned upside down, she was determined to put the cancer conversation on the airwaves too. When she approached me to work with her, I jumped at the chance. Who was this ballsy blonde woman who had twisted the arms of the BBC to run a podcast without so much as a pilot episode?

In her effort to talk candidly about living with cancer, Rachael put her faith in me and Lauren Mahon, two totally inexperienced broadcasters. Our podcast, You, Me and the Big C, was born. Each week, we would discuss our lives with the disease and our deepest fears. No topic was off limits. After our first recording, we knew we had created something special.

The success of the podcast and the thousands upon thousands of messages of support blew us away. We had reached number two in the iTunes chart, but were desperate for the top slot. On Tuesday 4 September, the day before Rach died, we did it. We got there and she was delighted. Rachael's mission has been accomplished: cancer is happening on prime time.

Since Rachael's death I've gone into overdrive talking about and remembering her. She made it easy to know what to do because she talked about her own mortality. For me, the big moment was our podcast with the actor Greg Wise, who cared for his sister Clare as she died from breast cancer. During that chat Rachael dictated her wishes (which included me wearing Gucci sunglasses and a big, black, floppy hat to her funeral) and her blueprint for how to live once she had gone. Make the most of every second, she ordered. If she could do that when dying, we must do so when granted the gift of living. We knew she would want us to carry on living, but to take her with us.

Death is my biggest fear, but Rach forced me to acknowledge it: to talk frankly about our hopes and our fears. Of course Rach didn't have a choice in how her cancer would play out, but she flipped the things she could control into something incredible. She could never accept not seeing her gorgeous son Freddie grow up, but knew she could control what she left him. Her drive to finish a book for him, a guide to life, kept her going.

As for me, I've already outlived my prognosis. On paper, I have an 8 per cent chance of making it to five years and I'm already two years in. I've had tumours taken out of my bowel, seven removed from my lungs and I'm about to embark on new treatment because my cancer has decided to wrap itself around an artery. I was meant to die first.

My heart breaks writing about Rachael and I'm really scared that I will follow next. However, I know I need to continue to talk about dying. I need to make people listen, not only to help me, but for them to know what to do. By bravely addressing her death, Rach allowed those close to her, especially her wonderful husband, to get on with living after she had gone.

Rach remembered Frank Sinatra in her final tweet posted on 3 September 2018: I'm afraid the time has come, my friends. Sadly, yes it has, my darling friend. But girl, you did it your way – with dignity, class and style. In your own words, you were, and always will be, terminally fabulous!

Lauren Mahon

Oh Freddie, where do I even start?

Mummy got in touch with me in December 2017 to submit a piece to my cancer community, GIRLvsCANCER, called 'The Fear'. Mummy wrote with a dry humour I'd come to absolutely adore. It was during these email exchanges that Mummy floated the idea of a 'cool cancer-blogging girls' podcast to me. 'Would I like to be involved?' Mummy asked.

We got busy plotting our episode topics, excitedly brainstorming our ideal guests and before you could say 'scanxiety' there we were with the wonderful Deborah James of BowelBabe, huddled around microphones in a BBC 5 Live studio recording *You, Me and the Big C*.

I'm in stitches remembering our recording of 'About Dating and Intimacy', our most requested podcast to date. As I was the only singleton of the trifecta, Mummy and Deb were determined to get me a good guy and even gave me my very own hashtag to begin the search. I really miss Mummy's perfectly timed inappropriate jokes so much.

We joked a lot, Freddie. We often laughed that we chatted about cancer like it was an episode of *EastEnders*. But that was the entire point. To open up the dialogue around the disease. Being open and honest and raw. To create a better understanding of the cancer experience to ensure that future Deborahs, Laurens and Mummys would never feel lost or alone. We were just three friends talking cancer taboos over a cup of tea. There just happened to be microphones in the room.

Since Mummy died we've been overwhelmed with the outpouring of love for both her and the podcast. And I couldn't be more proud! Messages confirming that Mummy's crusade to normalize the conversation around cancer is truly taking effect, that cancer patients are finding solace in our weekly chinwags, that carers are gaining an improved insight into what their loved ones are going through. And most importantly – Mummy would buzz off this – that the podcast is enabling medical practitioners to better treat their patients.

It's bittersweet though, Freddie. Because the only reason all this amazing stuff has happened, that the cancer conversation is centre stage, that people are beginning to sit up and listen – is Mummy. It's all your mummy.

The darkness left in the wake of your mummy's death is lit by the impressive legacy she has created. Mummy changed so many lives for the better. Including mine.

Mummy taught me the meaning of courage and class. She offered me a space on the podcast that became my very own sanctuary. My purpose. I'll be forever grateful for the role Mummy played in beginning to heal my broken heart.

It's strange getting back into that studio with your mum's seat bare. To not make her a brew or hand over my fan when it would be her turn to have a hot flush. I miss Mummy cooing over my latest purchase or cackling over inappropriate suggestions for GIRLvsCANCER slogans.

As per Mummy's wishes, Deb and I promise to continue with the podcast and I'm more determined than ever to continue the conversation Mummy started and to make you and Daddy proud. Your mummy is a rockstar, Freddie. Truly. I promise to keep her light shining bright in all the work that I do and to be there whatever you and Daddy need.

I'll love your mummy for ever. I'll be proud of her for always. And I am eternally grateful that Mummy let me be a part of her world.

Mike Holt

Freddie, in January 2018 I was asked by Rozina Breen at BBC 5 Live to talk to your mum about an idea she had about doing a podcast for people who have or have had cancer. Your dad and mum had been working on it at home. I was just going for a chat, but after five minutes she made me want to produce it and, luckily, she was really pleased when I asked to be her producer. Together we set about shaping the idea to make it work as a podcast. Quite simply, it is the most important piece of work I have ever had the privilege to be a part of.

We went through a list of people to be co-presenters and at the top of that list were the fantastic Deborah James and Lauren Mahon who were delighted to be asked. The four of us had a conference call and from the first few minutes I knew we had something special. Which is exactly what I told your mum when she phoned me afterwards. We called the show *You, Me and the Big C*. It was funny, emotional and, most importantly, a great source of help for people out there with cancer or who have a loved one who has it. Both you and your dad were a massive part of the pod. You were both always the most important thing to her.

Personally, working so closely with your mum was just a joy. She had so much to deal with at the time, but she was eternally positive, never once complaining and she had this amazingly wicked sense of humour that never failed to make me laugh. I will always be immensely proud to have helped bring her vision to reality. Also, to witness all three of them having such fun making this show, and for your mum to have a platform to shine alongside Debs and Lozza like never before, underlining the fantastically talented broadcaster she was. She sent me a message a few days before she died, telling me how proud she was, and that will always be very, very special to me. I will be forever grateful to be able to call her my friend.

When we first started, I think some people thought 'Who'd want to listen to a podcast about cancer?', imagining it might be a bit depressing. But the response from listeners from all around the world was so positive regarding the girls' honesty and humour when they talked about their experiences with cancer. The reaction to it blew us all away. Even Rachael was taken aback by the number of messages!

On the day before she died, your mum saw her podcast reach number one in the UK's iTunes charts. In October 2018, *You, Me and the Big C* was named Best New Show/Podcast at the UK's Audio and Radio Industry Awards (ARIA). The numbers of people that have downloaded and listened to the show is truly staggering. The pod team

– Deborah, Lauren, Al and I – are all so proud to have been a part of it, but this will always be your mum, Rachael's, legacy. She was a truly amazing person and has helped to change the way we talk about cancer. The outpouring of emotion when she died from people who never met her is testament to that. And you should be very proud, mate.

Alex Entwistle

Rachael was undeniably unique and a truly amazing person. Working with her, Debs, Lauren and Mike on the *You, Me and the Big C* podcast is one of the most rewarding and privileged jobs I've had in over fifteen years at the BBC. She brought us all together to work on something very, very special – a podcast that has helped, and will continue to help, more people than we could have ever imagined – and to be part of that is something I'll be eternally grateful for.

The ultimate professional as a newsreader, Rachael was serene and unshakeable, no matter how big or fast-moving the story. Beyond the microphone, she had a fantastically devilish sense of humour, perfectly countered by a mischievous laugh and angelic smile.

One of the many things I'll remember is the glow that appeared whenever she spoke about 'precious Freddie' and her husband Steve. Her love and admiration for those two was clear for everyone to see. Here's to a one-off and a true inspiration.

Chris Stark

Freddie, it is an honour to be even asked to say a few words about your incredible mum. I sadly never got to meet Rachael, as I was just a listener of the brilliant podcast that Rachael, Lauren and Deborah hosted. It was (and still is) so special and has helped a lot of people through the hardest part in their lives, and the lives of family members affected.

I had the tiniest of all roles of everyone who has written about your mum here. I was just a fan of the podcast when I was having a chat with its producer, Mike Holt, one night while travelling back from work. He told me that it would mean the world to your family if the podcast could get to number one in the charts. I saw that it was my one opportunity to chip in with something that could help to support the podcast that had supported so many people, so I got to work.

I sent messages to anybody and everybody on social media. Those who followed me, those who didn't, asking them to spread the word about the podcast and to start a bit of a campaign to get it to number one. People were so up for the challenge, of course they were; your mum had inspired everyone to get behind it. The very next day I woke up to a message from Mike saying it had reached number one. I heard that your mum smiled when your dad told her that.

We all hope to have a little impact on this world, in the short time we are here. Your mum did that and more. She showed how to face adversity with courage, confront sadness with happiness and with the number-one podcast she moved the front line of the war against cancer to a public place for everyone to rally behind. You must be so, so proud. All my best, always.

Emma Agnew

'You must meet Rachael, she's got cancer too.' Not exactly the introduction anyone would wish to hear. But, typical of your mum, she got in touch with me and so a friendship started. We both worked for the BBC, we were both in the breast-cancer club and we had both decided to 'go public' with our disease.

We chatted about all sorts of things: work; you, Freddie; and my children, Charlotte and Tom. We both loved horses, and I encouraged your mum to ride again when she went away to Scotland for her birthday (*very* much against doctor's orders!). We gassed on about all the wonderful holidays she wanted to take you on and the lovely sporting events we both enjoyed, like Wimbledon where we could get really dressed up in glamorous outfits. Oh, we did love shopping for clothes! We talked about our treatments; she opted for the cold cap during chemo and kept her glorious blonde locks, while I went cold turkey and had my hair shaved off. We checked in with each other when we knew we had scans due or important appointments. We encouraged each other when the steroids and drugs played havoc with our bodies, and we met for lunch and laughed. A lot.

We also wondered why my husband, Jonathan, and your dad, Steve, wouldn't address the 'what if?' issue at all. Was it all the 'hunter gatherer/man is protector' image? Or were they just too scared to look to a future without us? After all, would they ever be able to find anything ever again if we weren't around?! Then your mum and her amazing podcast team decided to do an episode on how our nearest and dearest coped with living with us and our cancer. It was a stroke of genius. With your dad hosting the programme, a husband, father and brother opened up to each other about what it's really like living with someone they love who has a life-threatening illness. While the patient is surrounded by the bubble of a medical team all doing everything in their power to keep us alive, our 'carers' are left on the sidelines. Jonathan confessed he found that very difficult, as his own life as a professional cricketer-turned-commentator means *he* is usually the centre of attention.

The broadcast really helped Jonathan and me be more honest with each other during those long months of treatment and, more importantly, we know that the men opening up helped so many thousands of others who were in the same situation. The feedback, love, support and sharing of similar stories was overwhelming. So, thank you, Rachael, for being so determined to get us all talking about – and living with – cancer. I'm lucky enough to be in remission and every time I take my horse for a ride across the glorious Leicestershire countryside, I think of my beautiful, generous friend, who was your adoring mum, and how she made living with cancer just that little bit more manageable for us all.

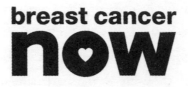

breast cancer now

MAKING LIFE-SAVING RESEARCH HAPPEN

We are incredibly humbled that with every sale of this book a portion of the proceeds are being donated to Breast Cancer Now, to support our work and help to make life-saving research happen.

Rachael was passionate about research and it is stories like hers that inspire us to keep making the discoveries and searching for the breakthroughs that will change the future of breast cancer, for ever.

Our world-class research focuses entirely on breast cancer and with nearly 380 scientists across the UK and Ireland, working on over 85 cutting-edge projects, we are tackling this devastating disease from every angle. From discovering how to prevent breast cancer and uncovering better ways to detect it earlier, to finding new ways to treat it and understand how to stop it spreading to other parts of the body – we won't stop until breast cancer has taken its last life.

We believe that if we all act now, by 2050, everyone who develops breast cancer will live – and live well. And for every life that is lost until we reach that day, like Rachael's, we are filled with a greater resolve and more determination to turn our vision into reality.

Thank you to the Bland family and everyone who has bought Rachael's memoir for their generous and incredible support.

TO FIND OUT MORE ABOUT OUR WORK, PLEASE GO TO
breastcancernow.org